Healthy *Stories*

Dedicated to the limited number of Public Health Servants and to the vast number of those who serve Public Health,

And to the Editors' and Authors' families.

ISBN: 978-0-615-61129-7
Copyright 2012.
Printed on recycled paper.
Printed in the United States of America.

Disclaimer:
The views and opinioins expressed in this journal are those of the authors alone and do not necessarily reflect the official policy, views, opinions or position of the Miami-Dade County Health Department or the State of Florida Department of Health. The Miami-Dade County Health Department is not responsible for the accuracy of any information supplied by the authors of *Healthy Stories*. Many of the stories are partially or totally fictional and any similarity to any person living or dead is merely coincidental.

Subscriptions:
Healthy Stories is published annually. Individual subscription rates are $11.00/year. Healthy Stories Editions 2007, 2008, 2009, 2010 and 2011 are available for $11.00 per issue. Prices include shipping and handling.

Healthy *Stories*

Illuminating the Human Condition

EDITOR-IN-CHIEF
Morton Laitner

SENIOR EDITORS
Philip Reichert
Amy Tejirian
Tracie L. Dickerson

ASSOCIATE EDITORS
Roland R. Pierre
Ninfa Urdaneta
J.D. Shingles
Heather Beaton
Frederick Villari
Frank Menendez
Caroline Glick
Samantha Feanny
Ben Zipken
Sam Gonas
Lauren McGurk

TRANSLATORS
Ninfa Urdaneta
Roland Pierre
Frank Menendez
Francisco Menendez

ASSISTANTS TO EDITORS
Gertrude Pendleton
Lorena Raschio

TECHNICAL SUPPORT
Suleydi SanMartin
Otto Rodriguez

Our Mission

Promoting and protecting health through stories

Our Vision

Creating a world-class, public health literary journal

Our Goals

To delight our readers
through laughter, tears and thought;

On how their health and health departments
affect their well-being;

While coaching book lovers on the art of story-telling
as the principal method to get their message heard,
understood and remembered;

Inspiring readers to write their health experiences for others
to make a personal connection with their own lives;

While always remembering not to take ourselves too seriously
and that humorous stories make the best medicines.

Contents

TRANSLATIONS

FOREWORD

From the Administrator of the Miami-Dade County Health Department

As Healthy Stories celebrates its sixth anniversary, I am proud to announce a new historical section in this volume. Cicero defines history as "the witness that testifies to the passing of time. It illumines reality, vitalizes memory, provides guidance in daily life and brings us tidings of antiquity." This year's compilation successfully meets Cicero's definition through one book and one website where our history is available to our world-wide readers.

Our public health past comes alive directly through the eyes, ears and mouths of the leaders of the Florida Department of Health. We are honored by the contributions of E. Charlton Prather, MD, MPH; M. Rony Francois, MD, MSPH, PhD; James T. Howell, MD, MPH; Robert M. Brooks, MD, MBA, MPH; and Ana M. Viamonte Ros, MD; five former Secretaries/Surgeon General of the agency. They shared how they handled crises, moved the department forward and fought to fulfill their mission of protecting and promoting health in Florida. Healthy Stories fulfills the important mission of creating an institutional memory. These eye-witness accounts allow us to find and explore our roots. I would to thank D. Russell Jackson, Jr., the Senior Vice President of the Florida Medical Association for writing the forward to this portion of our book.

Further, we have included two stories memorializing the late Dr. Carl Brumback who was known as "The People's Doctor" in Florida.

Healthy Stories continues to partner with South Florida Writers Association. For the past two years we have coproduced and sponsored the Mango Writers Conference, a conference where over one hundred authors and poets meet at the health department to sharpen their writing skills while focusing on the subject of health.

In addition, we continue to mentor Barry University's Masters Program students in the Bio-Medical, Occupational Therapy and

Health Sciences Administration programs. We are honored to present many of these students' works in this Healthy Stories volume. They give us a youthful outlook on modern day issues.

Stories in this volume focus on the following significant public health issues: bioterrorism, pregnancy and child birth, sexually transmitted diseases, alcoholism, depression, dieting, anorexia, obsessive–compulsive disorder, steroids and methamphetamine use, cancer and chemotherapy, prostate issues and PSA screening, dental health, strokes and high blood pressure, heart disease, and Alzheimer's.

I am proud that this edition of Healthy Stories honors Cicero as well as providing guidance for a healthy life through the art of story telling.

I hope you enjoy our literary journal.

Lillian Rivera,
R.N., M.S.N., Ph.D.

Introduction

Six years and running – our story book keeps on growing. Our publication has become a fixture in the public health world, filling a niche as the nation's one and only public health literary journal.

Our stories continue to charm, entertain, and touch the hearts of our readers. These gripping tales resonate authenticity. Many evoke OMGs from the mouths of our readers and bring tears to their eyes. Many present challenging choices which illustrate how to protect and preserve health.

Our editors search out vignettes that confront reality and illuminate the human condition. This year's edition returns to universal themes: forgiveness and redemption, living with a disability, charity, grief, and love.

Our authors are apt students of human nature. Many overcome their fears and display courage by putting their inner most feelings on paper.

Our readers inform us about how emotionally charged they have become after reading our book and how they have taken away many of life's lessons.

Wondrous Occurrences:
One of our authors, Liz Brady, delivered a copy of Healthy Stories to Clarence Clemons, the tenor saxophonist of Bruce Springsteen's E Street Band, as he lay dying in his hospital bed. The Big Man was appreciative saying, "Thanks," as he tightly held onto our book.

Getting an email from sound artist, Jim Green, thanking us for our story about his sound art in the Fort Lauderdale International Airport.

Doing a street reading from Healthy Stories on Miami Beach during Sleepless Night, a bi-annual all-night arts festival.

A quote from a public health nurse, "I have read all your stories online and they are so well written I consider them literature."

Listening to Healthy Stories radio as our authors read their tales.

Hearing from professors and classroom teachers who have published in Healthy Stories how they gained credibility with their students when they showed off the book.

Seeing how other websites, such as HowtoLoseWeight360.com, incorporate our stories as successful examples for their readership.

Receiving an email from Cairo, Egypt inquiring about the Mango Writers Conference

A professor of journalism at Boston's Northeastern University contacted us to find out how to reach Julie-Goldsmith-Gilbert, who was last year's keynote speaker at the Mango Writers Conference. He was doing research on her relative, Pulitzer Prize Winning author Edna Ferber.

We're amazed in our journal's cultural pervasiveness: Springsteen, Edna Ferber, Egypt, literature and radio. Wondrous!

Making a Difference in Our Community:
Awarding our book to the winners of the Junior Orange Bowl Creative Writing Contest.

Providing Healthy Stories to the Monroe County Health Department Environmental Staff, the Southeast Consortium of Health Department and Children's Medical Services, at the Grand Re-opening of the Penalver Clinic, to the Jefferson Reaves Clinic's Board of Directors, to representatives of the Afro-American Delegation of Dade County, the Miami-Dade Clerks of Court Office Eleventh Judicial District Probate Division, and to the Monroe County Commission.

Providing a copy to a Peace Corps stationed in Malawi, Africa.

Producing and cosponsoring, with the South Florida's Writer's Association, the Second Annual Mango Writers Conference that was held on the grounds of the Miami-Dade County Health Department and where attendees were invited to write Healthy Stories.

Law students for the University of Miami, St. Thomas University, Nova Southeastern University, Florida International University, University of Florida, and Stetson University helped edit Healthy Stories.

New Libraries Possessing Our Journal:
Pinecrest Library, Pinecrest, Pinecrest, Florida
Barry University Library, Miami Shores, Florida
University of South Florida Medical School Library, Tampa, Florida
Escambia County Library, Pensacola, Florida
Leon County Library, Tallahassee, Florida
Florida State University Library, Tallahassee, Florida
Palatka Library, Palatka, Florida
Key West Library, Key West, Florida
The Society of the Four Arts Library, Palm Beach, Florida
St. Thomas Law School Library, Miami, Florida
University of Miami School of Ethics Library, Coral Gables, Florida
Florida International University English Department Library, Miami, Florida
Bay County Library, Panama City, Florida

By the Numbers:
21,000 views on healthystories.net.
6,000 hard copies of Healthy Stories printed
$33.12 highest price ever asked for a Healthy Stories book on EBay
1200 people receive our stories via email
550 websites reference Healthy Stories
400 stories and poems are published on healthystories.net
160 submissions received for this edition 60 accepted
150 total number of authors published in our books
90 attendees at the Second Annual Mango Writers Conference
75 stories translated and published in Spanish and Creole

20 staff members worked on this edition of Healthy Stories

6 editions of Healthy Stories

6 years of being number 1 on Google search results when searching Healthy Stories

5 years we sold books at the Miami International Book Fair

3 books given to each published author

1 Healthy Stories volume out of circulation (2007 edition)

Publicity:

The Florida Journal of Public Health, Spring/Summer 2011 Issue 207 a reprint of "A Survivors Love Story" by John Holmes

Reflections, the Magazine of Southern University Law Center, Winter 2010 Volume 21 Number 1

The South Florida Writer's Association's monthly newsletter, Author's Voice

Miami-Dade County Health Department's E-HealthBeat Fall/ winter 2011

The Medical Books Center, www.echocardiology.org

We hope our stories will illuminate your human condition by bringing good health into your lives.

The Editors

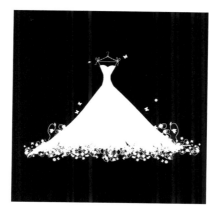

Don't Get Your Hopes Up

By Tracie Dickerson

As I stood out on our balcony, staring at the crystal blue ocean, the world trembled around me. I grabbed a chair to steady myself. My stomach lurched and I felt faint. When my knees stopped shaking, I walked back into the room and over to Rich.

"Mvywsnifflemwomxsiqntphvehiomslpbizaulsniffleduorcyto-borstyhliwnksihrewlolodpive," I wailed. After a few more tries, I eventually was able to get out the message, and we packed up our room.

———

Ninety days ago I got engaged in Aruba. But this is not the story of what lead up to my engagement, but instead it is the story of what happened afterward. It started innocently enough, as many stories do. It started when I called my mom to tell her of my exciting news.

In a panicked tone, my step-dad Larry answered, "Tracie, I'm glad you called. We've been trying to find you all day."

My first thoughts were "Wow! I guess Rich, my fiancé called them – they must be so happy. Why didn't mom answer?"

Larry's voice cracked as he said, "Your mom is in critical condition in

ICU, the doctors think it is best if you come to see her and say goodbye."

I, a woman of many words, lost mine. This was supposed to be one of the happiest moments of my life, and I had been dealt a huge blow to the gut. "I'll be there as soon as I can, but don't get your hopes up that I will be there tomorrow... not every island has a flight every day, and all of tonight's flights have left."

Larry sobbed, "I hope you won't be too late."

My happy message about the wedding went undelivered.

Rich and I learned the fastest way to Houston was to fly back to Miami. The next morning we arrived at the airport and found out the airline changed our flight without notification. We missed our plane. Panic set in, and I freaked out. We were sent to the airline office, and after an hour were told nothing could be done. All the flights for Sunday were booked, and we shouldn't get our hopes up about flying standby.

In a moment of clarity, I noticed the monitors listed one last flight from Aruba to Miami, leaving in under an hour on American Airlines. My stomach quivered. I had high hopes as I walked to the counter and began my tale of woe. I tried hard to keep my crying under control, but as fears of missing another flight and thoughts of not being available to hold my mom's hand as she died washed over me, Rich stepped in and within a few minutes, we were going home. Rushing through security and onto the plane, I prayed for my mom.

I arrived in Miami and immediately left for Texas. I rushed straight to the ICU, to see my mom. Again I cried. At first I cried because I was so relieved to see her. Then I cried because I saw her. I saw her feeding tubes, I saw her fourteen IVs, I saw her monitors, I saw the cooling pad for her fever, and I saw her life support breathing machine. Then I cried because of what I didn't see – her eyes were open, but there was no sparkle, her mouth was open, but there was no smile. Her hands were warm, but she couldn't hold mine. She did not know I was there.

I cried and cried and cried. For all the lost moments, for all the lost opportunities, for all the things we never said but should have, for all the things that she would miss out on. For never getting to see her daughter married, for never getting to meet her grandchildren. I cried for a long time the first night, and when I was done I decided to make every last moment count. My mom was heavily sedated.

A nurse explained, "She is in a medically induced coma that allows the body to heal, without putting the patient in distress."

During my first night at the hospital her odds of survival were very low. Everyone, but me, was waiting for her to die.

On the morning of the second day I started my new routine. There were six hourly visits allowed per day. My new routine included four hours of sleep followed by sixty minutes with my mom, a drive to the hotel, a quick bite of breakfast, ninety minutes of sleep, then back to the hospital for an hour with my mom, then three hours for myself, rinse and repeat.

My first few hours alone with her were unbearable. Each doctor I saw found a new way to relay the worst case scenario. To them, my mother was a science project. They no longer saw a person, only a way to advance the field of medicine. I chose to read to my mom, just like she did with me. I read out loud and painstakingly described each and every detail of the giant stack of bridal magazines I purchased. I described the dresses with all the detail and fervor a tomboy could... "This one looks like something run through the shredder and then sewn onto a garbage bag.... This one looks like it needs some serious ironing. And my personal favorite, here's one that looks like a swan got hot glued to the skirt." I read and I read hoping something got through.

As the days passed, my mom and I planned out my wedding. She never complained about my crazy ideas, my thoughts about pricing, the guest list and the seating chart. "A big destination wedding," I said, "with five hundred people. I want barbeque, a giant cake, horse drawn carriages, and a shrimp extravaganza – like Bubba Gump – even an ice sculpture shaped like a shrimp!" Most mothers-of-the-Bride would have fainted at the mere thought. But my mom kept her cool. She laid there blissfully unaware of the decisions I was making. Her monitors beeped and her life support system continued at a steady pace as I picked out her champagne colored dress, my dad's tuxedo, and created a Cajun menu complete with mudbugs.

One morning I walked into her room and she had one less tube, and the next time she was down another. A few more tubes gone and the doctors determined it was time to "wake her up." They removed the sedation. As I held her hand, I hoped to feel something twitch, some signal my mom was still in there. As the hours ticked by, my mom remained unresponsive.

The doctors said, "It is highly likely your mother is brain dead… at this point people who are removed from sedation should have some sort of response." They poked, they prodded, they had saved her body, but they were unable to save her. To them, their science project failed. I was the one in shock. As the only relative present, I would have to relay the message to my family.

After the doctor left, my favorite nurse came over and hugged me. "I see this a lot," she said, "give your mama some more time. Some people don't get up right away, some folks just take a lil' bit longer."

The nurse was right. My mom became so aware of her surroundings she was put back on sedation to keep her calm while she healed. As she began to get better, I made my way back to Miami. As my mom entered the rehab hospital, my family was told she may never be able to walk again. The family got together and renovated her house. We worked and worked, removing furniture, ripping out carpet, widening doorways, putting down the wood floors she had always wanted and generally getting ready for her return. Over the course of the next few weeks, my mom defied the doctor's predictions. Within thirty days she went from nearly dead to fully alive. After not hearing her voice in over forty-five days, she surprised me with her first phone call.

"Whatcha doin'?" she said.

I looked around my office and the piles of work and replied, "Not too much. What are you up to?"

"Just strollin' around the hospital with my walker." I laughed as I thought about how sore my arms were after all of the hard work we put in at her house, and how much she will appreciate the cold winter ahead when she walked on her new floors.

Ninety days later my mom and I continued our discussion about the wedding. I explained that I had gone over all of the details with her already, and she had agreed because she never objected. When I got to the part about the ice sculpture in the shape of a giant shrimp, she simply replied, "Don't get your hopes up!" ☼

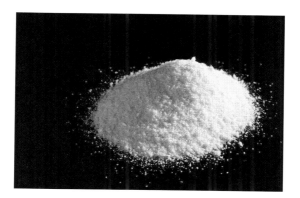

The Drums of Ether

By Mort Laitner

R ing, Ring, Ring, I picked up the receiver. "Good morning, Legal Department, how may I help you?"

"Hi, I'm the principal of Homestead Elementary School. I need your help. Two days ago the Miami-Dade Police Department raided a cocaine laboratory that is located one block away from my school. They arrested the owner of the house and the coke lab's criminal chemists. Did you read the story in yesterday's Miami Herald?"

"I've read numerous articles in the Herald about cocaine cowboys, major drug busts, and even attorneys losing their licenses for abusing the substance. But, I haven't heard about this coke lab next door to a school," I replied.

The principal continued, "About a week ago, I drove past that house and I smelled ether. I'll never forget that nauseating sweetish smell because when I was a kid, I had my appendix removed. The anesthesiologist put me under using ether. I thought those doctors were trying to gas me to death. I'm no Sherlock Holmes but that pungent odor—my nose told me that the bad guys were processing cocaine. I read how it was manufactured, or do they say 'processed,' in Newsweek. So I called the police and suggested that they put the house under surveillance and get a search and seizure warrant. Boy was I right! The cops confiscated baggies full of coke. Who knows what the street value of that stuff was."

"I don't have a clue," I replied. "I thought the cops did a great job until I personally inspected the premises and saw forty ether-filled metal drums. The property now is a hazardous waste dump. They used ether to process that toxic stuff."

As the principal spoke, I wondered, "How is this a public health emergency?" Having never been to a coke lab, my curiosity got the best of me.

The principal continued, "I don't know if you're aware of it, but ether is flammable, volatile, and a highly explosive substance. I've seen a number of fifteen-year-old scavengers hanging out at this coke lab. I've also seen these same teenagers smoking cigarettes as they rummage through the property. Now, I fear those dumb cigarette-smoking kids will light up near those drums. Did you know the ether fumes are colorless?"

I shook my head to myself, indicating I had no clue.

"One flicker of flame and the coke lab explodes and my school will be blown to smithereens. We have over 200 students and 20 staff members at Homestead Elementary," said the principal.

"Sir, let me assure you that I am going to give this matter my highest priority. I have to research the law to determine the health department's authority to handle this case. I've got to draft and file pleadings with a criminal court judge, the state attorney, and the public defender asking the court's permission to have these drums of ether hauled away."

The principal sighed in relief, "Thanks for working on this project. I don't want my students or teachers to die. Please keep me posted as to your actions. Here's my phone number."

I proceeded to do the research and determined that these cocaine cowboys had created a sanitary nuisance that threatened the health and lives of children and staff. I drafted a search and seizure warrant authorizing the Miami-Dade County Health Department to enter the property, seize the drums of ether, and properly dispose of them. As I dictated the pleading to my secretary, I wondered if I would see any cocaine on the premises.

This is what I told the judge: "Your Honor, the Miami-Dade County

Health Department is here today to protect the lives of over 200 children and 20 staff members housed at Homestead Elementary School. There is a potentially explosive situation on our hands, one that could blow the roof off an elementary school. Next door to the school there are 40 drums of ether with each drum holding up to 55 gallons. The drums of ether were left abandoned in a busted coke laboratory. I need your permission and an order to have these highly explosive canisters of ether removed from this former drug lab and safely placed in an area where children's lives will not be harmed."

The judge asked, "Counselor, do you have a warrant ready for my signature?"

I said, "Your honor, I do," as I approached the bench and handed the judge the order.

She examined the document and asked, "Mr. Public Defender, do you have any objections to the issuance of this warrant for the seizure and disposal of these drums?"

"No, your honor, my clients have no objection," the public defender replied.

"Ms. Assistant State Attorney, do you have any objection to these drums being confiscated by the health department and disposed of prior to going to trial?"

The assistant state attorney responded, "No objection your honor."

As the judge signed the warrant, she expressed her appreciation, "I want to personally thank the health department for taking on this serious problem and protecting the lives of these children."

As I left the court room, I was accompanied by an environmental health worker named Thorn. As I gripped the court order in my hands, Thorn looked me straight in the eyes and snorted, "Wipe that victory smile off your face. This wasn't the trial of the century."

"Thorn, you're absolutely right. But, save your comments for someone who cares. We have to figure out how to wrap this case up."

After calling numerous hauling companies, we found one willing to pick up and clean out the drums at no cost—in exchange for ownership of the drums. We arranged to meet the hauling company at the site.

As Thorn drove me to the coke lab, I again wondered if we would see any cocaine.

As we walked in the partially destroyed laboratory, I said, "Thorn, it is really an interesting set up. It reminds me of chemistry in high school with the Bunsen burners, the beakers and the baking trays."

With his lips shut Thorn pointed with his index finger to a baking tray containing small quantities of coke buried in its crevices. "You know what that is?" he queried.

"Yeah, that's cocaine! Why didn't the cops destroy it?"

I continued to inspect the building. Thorn stayed in the room with the coke samples. A few minutes later Thorn joined me as we watched the haulers lift the last of the metal drums onto the 18-wheeler semi. I pondered if he had tasted the coke, but did not ask.

Alone, I reentered the lab, walked over to the baking tray, and scraped my finger across the white powder. Slowly I moved my index finger toward my nose while staring at the substance. Then I flicked the coke into the air and watched it snow down. As the flakes floated toward the floor, I breathed a sigh of relief as a victory smile gripped my face. ☼

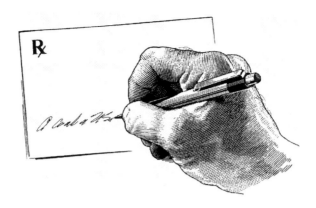

Cascade

By Stefanie Sveiven

The pain was like an unrelenting mosquito ignoring constant swats of irritation, a nuisance. As I assaulted the source of the pain with my prodding tongue, the hygienist's warning from a few months prior found my ear again.

"It's going to be difficult to keep those teeth clean back there. You need to get those extracted."

Time made sport of teasing me and it was constantly running away like a playful three year old. I had too many things to do and not enough time to commit to surgery and have these wisdom teeth removed. I didn't want the chipmunk cheeks and I couldn't afford to be out of commission, if even for a few days.

"They grew in just fine," I assured myself, noting that they did actually fit in my mouth. But truthfully, the lower two wisdom teeth had an umbrella of gum partially covering where the teeth met the back of my mouth.

Again, I probed the inflamed mound of gum covering my lower right wisdom tooth with my tongue. Opening my mouth wide in front of the mirror, that bit of gum looked an angry red as it engulfed the intruding tooth. Space was limited. I sighed and pursed my lips in thought. I put it off long enough, I needed to see the dentist and get these teeth removed. Leaving my reflection behind in the restroom, I exited into the hallway. The nurse practitioner I work for saw me toying with my mouth.

"What's up, girl?" she asked.

I opened my mouth wide again and gestured towards the agitated area.

"Whoa," she remarked, "That's nasty." I closed my mouth in dismay. As if I had pressed the "Replay" button at the end of the YouTube video I just watched, I heard again, "You need to get those things removed, and soon. You don't want that to have an infection like that."

The "and soon" part of her remark prompted my usual cascade of ridiculous thoughts. If I didn't get them extracted soon, not only would that bothersome gum continue to suck the pleasure out of eating, but the infection could get worse. My mind, absolutely fascinated by cause and effect in the medical world, crafted a wild story of an intelligent, pre-med college student leaving her infected gum to fester into an infection of her tooth, and then to the mandible which would spread to her brain and kill her; a terrible and preventable end to such a bright future!

Feeling my boss's inquisitive eyes on me, I quickly removed myself from the exquisitely wrought mosaic of ridiculous details I assigned to my hypothetical death. I ventured back into reality just in time to hear my boss suggest a round of antibiotics to clear up the infection. After examining the cascade of events leading to my potential death, I quickly agreed to the prescription of Clindamycin. After all, I knew the maxillofacial surgeon wouldn't touch me until the infection was cleared up.

Following the prescription orders, I finished my ten day cycle of Clindamycin. The infected mound of gum, with all the gall to irritate and cause me pain for a few weeks, was quickly overpowered by the Clindamycin and relinquished its efforts to cause me misery.

Within a few days the gum receded to reveal the remaining half of my wisdom tooth, but it clung to the very edge of my tooth in waiting. I knew it would strike again, if given the opportunity. I was unaware that my health had a greater enemy than this little bit of gum, until abdominal pain, cramping and bloating made me hastily forget about my appointment to get my wisdom teeth removed. My days became peppered with frequent and urgent trips to the rest-room. The doctor in me inspected all that escaped my body with an observant eye. What I found each time in the toilet was frightening. Bright orange and red with a strange consistency. I feared that my intestines were falling apart. After a week and a half of hopeful confidence in the strength of my super-human immune system, I was only getting worse. Extreme exhaustion plagued me. My pro-ductivity metamorphosed into idleness. Having a habit of self-diag-nosis, I googled my symptoms for answers. Everything I typed in gave me one result, IBS or Irritable Bowel Syndrome. I called into a gastroenterologist office and pleaded for a same day appointment for Friday afternoon.

The cacophonous roar from the waiting room, like a deluge, filled the hall as I exited the elevator. I reached the office door and turned the knob to find innumerable patients. I waded to the front window to check in, and then I scanned the room hopeful to find a bathroom, just in case. I had no luck in finding a bathroom or a seat. So I stood, fingers crossed that my intestines could withstand the wait.

My exhaustion served as an escape from the yellow sea of pa-tients, and I say yellow as most of them were jaundiced, a result of their gastrointestinal ailments. I found myself in the deepest sleep one can manage with their eyes open until I heard my name called, three hours later. I was never more a lummox than following the nurse to the scale in all my tired stupor. I clumsily approached an-other recent enemy of mine. I had avoided the scale for months now, since finishing my last season of college volleyball. I replaced prac-tice and workout time with the sport of eating anything and every-thing. I became a gold-medalist in plate cleaning.

Stepping onto the scale, I looked straight forward as I heard the dreadful sound of the nurse sliding the big weight over a notch or two. Finishing with a movement of the smaller weight, the nurse called out a number that I did not expect to hear. Despite tripling my daily caloric intake for the past few months and abolishing any routine regarding physical activity, I managed to lose ten pounds! Initially titillated that I was not the fat cow I should be with my current eating habits, I quickly understood this weight loss was cer-tainly a reflection of the gravity of my illness over the last week and a half. I was sick enough to lose ten pounds in a little over a week. I was directed to the waiting room.

The doctor sauntered in and placidly asked, "So what's up with you?"

I already appreciated his relaxed manner as I was being seen or such an un-lady like condition. As a very observant pre-med student, I had mentally noted the duration of my illness, when it started, and descriptively and carefully listed off each of my symptoms to the doctor. I even offered up a photo of my freaky bowels that I took with my iPhone to send to my mom, to which she texted back "I'm not a poop expert." The doctor laughed at me, taken aback by my medical jargon and interest in presenting him with a photo of my 'findings.' He declined the photo of my visual stool sample with a chuckle. He asked if I was interested in becoming a doctor. I informed him that I was in a master's program and planning to continue on to med school and he nodded omnisciently.

Following the detailed descriptions I listed in response to his casual question, the doctor stated playfully, "Don't tell me, as a future doctor, you were just in Mexico drinking a bunch of water and now you came back and you feel all sick."

I laughed, "No way, Jose."

Like a detective, he mastered asking questions in a certain sequence in order to get all the answers he needed. As if crossing this first question off his usual list of questions, he rolled right into another, "Have you taken any antibiotics recently?"

Being the type of person who avoids all medication, even aspirin, I was eager to respond with a swift, "No." But just as I started to reply, I recalled my obtrusive wisdom tooth and all the pain it caused me. Clindamycin, like a knight in shining armor, fought that gum infection to the death and prevailed. Again, and as usual, my mind ventured out of the present and as I came back to realize the doctor awaiting my response, I blurted out "Clindamycin." I recounted the details of my gum infection and thus my prescription for Clindamycin which I finished up two weeks prior.

A broad smile found his face. "You're making this too easy," he said, "So you've been exhausted, more exhausted than ever before, you've had severe abdominal cramps, strange and frequent stool, and constant nausea. You just finished Clindamycin two weeks ago, and a week and a half ago you started noticing these awful symptoms." My eyes were wide with anticipation. With the same casualness as his first question he stated "You have C. diff, I'm sure of it." I waited three hours in the waiting room for him to come to a quick fifteen minute conclusion, it was remarkable.

He went on to explain that Costridium Difficile was a very small bacterium, unable to compete with the natural bacterial flora in my intestines. Upon taking a broad spectrum antibiotic, and specifically Clindamycin, the natural flora in my intestines was wiped out leaving the small C. diff bacterium to flourish. The bacterium is poisonous and pumped toxins into my body causing all of my symptoms. All I could focus on was the word "difficile" in the name. Though not fluent, after five years of taking and speaking Spanish, I certainly know difícil means difficult and that's not good news to me when I'm spending much of my day straddling a toilet. My hope that the end of my toilet struggles was near shattered upon my translation of difficile, and then buried deep into the ground when the doctor added, "C. diff is a real b****."

Crap. Literally and figuratively. The doctor informed me that this is becoming a very common diagnosis for him and that there is a game plan for treatment. According to him, there are nine steps in treating C. diff and I could be better at step one, or it might take all nine. So I began with step one, the antibiotic Flagyl.

I left the office happy to have a diagnosis, and hopeful that step one would do the trick. What the doctor did not tell me was that Flagyl was about to rock my world like an AC/DC concert. Still nauseated from C. diff itself, the addition of Flagyl (a symptom of which is extreme nausea) magnified my nausea. Flagyl cannot be taken on an empty stomach, a shame when nausea hit me so hard that ingesting food of any kind set off my gag reflex. Getting up in the morning, I felt like yesterday was my 21st birthday and that I had seen the bottom of many tequila bottles, but without all the fun of celebrating my birthday. And I awoke to no gifts! I had to take off from work and school. Working for nurses helped my cause, as they were well aware of my state of being with C. diff and Flagyl setting up a bivouac within my sasquatch body. They allowed me to work at my own pace and offered their support. I was slightly offended that even with my Viking stature, being Norwegian, I could be weakened by a measly bacterium and antibiotic. Stricken with anomie, I retired to my chambers for the major part of every day. You can imagine how much studying got done while I slept my life away.

For a total of three weeks, I was incapable of performing my duties as a student, tutor, lab assistant and programmer for the Campus Health Center. I was too tired to stay awake, too nauseated to get out of bed, and not potty-trained enough to be out of a bathroom's reach. I hit bottom. In the few moments I could stay awake I read about C. diff. I read that often patients feel like they're dying when they have C. diff, and I definitely agreed. But after two weeks of the worst of the worst, I began to notice I was getting better. My abdominal cramps, bloating and bowels were much better. My energy was still very poor, and I would chug a 5-hour Energy drink only to fall asleep moments later. Espresso became my before bed drink. The nurses I work for let me know that I was going to be exhausted for a while. But aside from the exhaustion, weird things began to happen.

I mastered language at a young age. I rarely made errors in writing or in speech growing up. My father, with his masters in English and love of words, never spoke to us as children but always as adults. He even altered our children's books when he read them aloud and inserted more suitable, adult words. We were expected to catch on to his 'big words.' I became as verbose as my father and was always teased for my clear and precise enunciation (especially with 't's as in 'buttons' or 'kittens'). So, when I began to slur my words and jumble my sentences, my friends and I took quick notice. Furthermore, being an athlete my entire life, it was easy to diagnose that my proprioception was way off. I was unaware of my limb's location and continued to hit my arms and legs on things and slam my hands in doors. My coordination was very poor. My bowels were finally lady-like again but now I was a speech impaired, uncoordinated, giant mess. I dragged my ungainly, six-feet-tall behind to the GI for my follow up.

Déjà-vu, the doctor's office was just as it was the first time, the same flood of faces and babbling voices. I was called back and weighed, still ten pounds lighter, and then sent to the room to wait for the doctor. When he entered he began his round of follow-up questions. He was happy to hear that his diagnosis was dead on. "Sometimes I'm wrong," he said superciliously. His tone suggested that by sometimes he meant once, at most. He could be as cocky as he wanted though. I wasn't imprisoned by the toilet anymore, so he did his job. I then proceeded to explain my new ineptitudes: the memory impairment, the slurred speech, the lack of coordination and proprioception, all my friends laughing at me and my degradation right before their eyes. I explained these things were very recognizable as they were definitely uncharacteristic of me. Of course, he knew the answer to this also.

"It's the Flagyl. Judging by how sick it made you, you're just experiencing the serious end of the side effects. Some people get numbness in their extremities and other neurological issues. Keep an eye on them, they should be gone within a few weeks."

Maybe my hypothetical situations of what could go wrong aren't that ridiculous after all. Perhaps rather than batting away the irritating mosquito, I should imagine it could bite me and give me malaria. I will squash it before it does. ☼

Stefanie Sveiven is a pre-med student in the biomed graduate program at Barry University in Miami Shores, Florida.

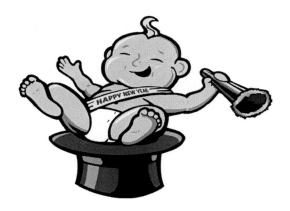

The Dump

By Samantha E. Feanny

ince childhood, I have always been told by my parents that I can do anything I want as long as I work really hard to get it. It seemed simple enough then and I have tried to keep it as a running theme throughout my life. I worked hard in high school, graduated with honors and got a scholarship to university. I did the same thing in university and again in law school. When it came time to find a job I felt that my perseverance had paid off. Never did I ever think, however, that my go-getter attitude would need to be applied to getting a man to poop in a hat.

It all started on a Friday morning. I woke up excited, not necessarily to go to another stunning day at work at the health department, but more because I was meeting my husband and sister at the airport that afternoon for a weekend getaway to Guatemala. As soon as I entered the main door to the office, however, I knew something was up.

My boss, Mort, had gathered all the troops he could find. They were sitting around the long conference table having some kind of heated discussion. I thought to myself, Staff meeting? No, Lorena (my administrative assistant) was fairly good at reminding me about those. Also, it had to be something big as the flipchart had been brought out and there was some kind of drawing on it that looked to me like a fast food king with minions at his feet.

Caroline, my co-worker, immediately shot me the "here we go again look" and I took a seat at the table. Mort didn't bother to stop and recap for me but eventually I got the gist of what had happened. Apparently, there was a family in Miami who may or may not have Typhoid Fever. The bigger problem was that one male family member worked for a restaurant and therefore posed a threat to the public.

As I listened to the discussion I started to piece together the main issues. Typhoid is a life-threatening illness, it is still common in many parts of the world, it is passed by shedding Salmonella Typhi bacteria, and the ickiest part . . . the shedding occurs through fecal matter. Our role was thus to protect the public by keeping the possible carrier out of the restaurant until he could be thoroughly tested.

We came up with a plan. We would draft an agreement to be signed by the man stating that he would not go to work until he was cleared. Someone from our office would accompany Dr. Conte, the head of our epidemiology department, and his team to the man's house, explain the situation and get him to sign. I thought this was a great idea as it would avoid the delay in getting a court order. All that needed to be decided was who would go.

I would like to say that I volunteered for solely altruistic reasons but that would not be entirely true. The way I saw it was I would go in with Frank, another attorney in our office, and Dr. Conte's team. "They would hand the man the agreement, he would sign it and I would get out a little early for my good deed and start my vacation. My delusion, however, was shattered when Mort turned to me and said quite sternly, "You are not to leave that house until you get the first sample."

I stared back at him blankly thinking to myself, sample? Nobody mentioned anything about a sample before I stuck my stupid hand up. He went on, "Dr. Conte says we need at least three samples and we can only get one every twenty-four hours so we need to make sure we get the first one now. I'm not taking any chances."

I shook my head and said in the most confident voice I could muster up, "Okay, I'm sure that won't be a problem. He'll just use the bathroom and I'll make sure they get it."

"No!" Mort exclaimed, "I want you to go in there and make sure no funny business goes down. You have to check the bathroom and make sure the sample we get isn't from someone else." At this point I just figured I had entered the twilight zone and nodded.

I left the office with the agreement and clear orders from Mort. I would go to a stranger's house, inspect his bathroom for imposter poop, ask him to poop in a hat-like container while I waited, and return with the signed agreement. I chuckled a bit while imagining what everyone's face would look like if I brought the sample back to the office instead of the agreement.

Frank and I arrived at the apartment complex at about 11:00 a.m. The team was waiting outside for us. We introduced ourselves as the lawyers and followed them to the home. At the front door, we were greeted by the man's older sister, her two kids, and her cousin. She explained in broken English that he was on his way home and that she had already threatened him that he better be here. We laughed, saying there was no need to threaten and that we were just there to help.

The home was too small for our entire team so Frank and I hung in the open air hallway of the building. When some of the others stepped out, I took the opportunity to do my little "inspection." There was thankfully no poop as yet. To this day I'm not really sure what I would have done if there were any rogue samples lying around.

The man arrived about ten minutes later, looking a bit shocked to find his home and hallway invaded by the health department. We introduced ourselves and to my dismay he stuck his hand out for us to shake. I'm not a rude person and I really hope he didn't see me cringe, but all I could think when I took his hand was Great, now I have Typhoid. We then worked through our thoroughly practiced script on why we were there, what the danger of Typhoid Fever was, and why we needed him to sign the agreement. Surprisingly, he took it all quite well, said he understood and signed. Then I broke the news to him.

I stood there in this stranger's house, looked him dead in the eye and said, "Thank you for being so cooperative but I need one more thing from you."

He looked a bit puzzled and asked, "What?"

I replied, "I'm going to need to get a sample from you today so can you please take this container and give us one?"

He stared at me again, "A sample of what?"

Things had now gone into that awkward stage I had been dreading all day. "Well," I said, "in order to make sure you don't have Typhoid we need to get three fecal samples so I really have to get one from you today."

"Oh," he said.

"I know, this is uncomfortable, but I really can't leave until you give us one."

"That might be a problem. This isn't my normal time and I don't think I'll be able to just go like that."

Feeling a bit frantic, I replied, "Maybe have some prunes or something? Coffee may do the trick. I'm sure we have some fruit. You want some granola?"

"I'm sorry, I just don't think this is going to happen. I promise I'll give them a sample though. I just can't do it right now."

I thought about it for a second and then I remembered my very clear instructions. "Look," I said, "I can't leave here without a sample. My boss will not be happy if we don't come back with your poop and I really don't like to be around him when he's unhappy. I'm begging you to just use the bathroom. I'll wait."

I'm not sure if it was the desperation in my voice or Frank's suggestions on things that help him do Number Two, but after about two hours of pleading in the hot windless hallway, we finally got our sample.

I returned to the office feeling quite triumphant that day. I didn't bring the poop in like I wanted to, but the signed agreement seemed to please Mort enough. So I guess the moral of this story is, if you work hard and spend at least two hours begging, you can get a total stranger to poop in a hat.

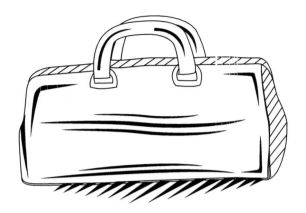

Sitting Shiva

By Mort Laitner

Three days after my Dad's death, I sat shiva in my mother's Boca Raton home. In her villa, a group of ten adults—our minyan—stood, talked and waited for the Rabbi to make his appearance.

Alone I stared out the kitchen's glass doors at the lake and the golf course. I flashed back at how happy my father was when Jason, his grandson, caught a large bass in that lake. I smiled realizing that picture had become one of my unerasable Kodak moments.

Each day of Shiva, I sipped flavorless coffee as my reddened eyes noticed that the lake appeared a paler shade of blue and the golf course a browner shade of green. I recalled the sweet taste and rich aroma of my Dad's freshly-brewed coffee. How it ran over my tongue and ignited my taste buds. How in this kitchen I sat looking at him and at this lake.

Walking into the living room, I found myself surrounded by acquaintances, family and unknown friends of my parents. My father had touched all their lives. They shook my hand, expressed their condolences and said how much they respected my Dad.

Lining the living room walls were impressionistic paintings. I scanned them and realized that they represented my blurred life. In this living room, on these couches, next to these paintings, my Dad and I talked for hours. He was a master storyteller--a male Scheherazade. We discussed wars, history and how life was treating us. He told off-color jokes and I laughed. I loved his sense of humor and he knew it. Those days and those laughs were now gone forever.

The Rabbi's appearance broke my day-dreaming. He instructed the minyan to stand and face east. He led us in prayer. He helped my Mom, my sister and I recite the Mourner's Kaddish. As the three of us searched for meaning and comfort in this spiritual ritual, I silently prayed: G-d walk through our house and take away our sorrow and please watch over us and heal my family.

After the Rabbi left the villa, two elderly men cornered me in the vestibule. "Hi, I'm Saul, and this is David. It is our pleasure to meet you."

They appeared to be in their late sixties or early seventies... short, balding men with protruding stomachs. They both wore white cotton short-sleeve shirts and like my father, bore tattooed numbers on their forearms. I shook their hands and glanced into their eyes. I sensed they were messengers, sent to tell me a story, sent to hand me another piece to the puzzle that made up my father's life.

In a thick Polish accent, Saul said, "You know you look an awful lot like your father."

"Thanks." I replied. "Many folks considered him a handsome man."

David piped in, "Many women loved the way he looked and dressed. He told us many stories about the time he spent in Rome--before the war, when he was in medical school---about those beautiful Italian women he knew. Boy, could he tell a story...so descriptive... down to the minutest detail."

Now Saul interrupted, "Your father befriended us during the last days of the war... in the death camp, just days before we were all liberated by the Soviet Army."

"We wanted to tell you that he saved our lives." David continued as he rubbed his tattoo.

I remembered hearing those words before. Usually from my father's patients or their family members who told me how he pulled them away from death and back to the living.

"Thanks for telling me. How did he do it?" I inquired as I pulled on the small piece of black cloth pinned to my jacket.

"He gave us the most important gift of all...the will to live," Saul said.

David continued, "Well it was near the end of the war. We were all imprisoned in a concentration camp...inches away from death. We were ill and starving. We were skin on bones. We heard the bombs exploding in the distance, but we didn't know how many days it would be before the Russian Army liberated us. Every minute, prisoners died all around us. Both of us were sixteen years old, and your father knew we were virgins. He kept telling us to keep struggling, not to give up on life, to stay alive because making love to women was something we had to experience. He told us one story after another about his sexual escapades."

As David talked, my mind wandered. "Did my Dad know that by telling these stories to these young men he was also saving his own life? Was storytelling his salvation---his medicine of hope and love? Would I exist if not for those stories?"

I observed tears forming in David's eyes as he whispered, "He kept our minds off of food and death. He gave us hope in our darkest moment. Your father, without medicines, used the only tool left in his medical bag...his brain."

Saul jumped in, "A brilliant strategy. It worked! We fought death and we won. I doubt that without those stories we would be talking to you today."

Hugging both of them, I replied, "Thanks so much for telling me your moving story. My Dad never did."

Alone I stared out the kitchen window, feeling proud of my Dad. I now noticed the brilliance of the lake's blue waters and the sharpness of the green radiating off the golf course. ☼

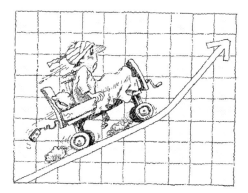

Frequent Flyer

By Robert Hill

D o you know that page of text that appears before a crime show on late night television? They usually state something about altering the names to protect the innocent. The following story deserves one of the pages. The names have been changed and places altered, but the events – as offensive as they are – are true.

"Hey John," Susan said smiling that devilish smile that meant the request was something that I would not want to do. "Can you do me another favor? Kevin is acting up in the lobby again."

I looked down the hall toward the doors to the emergency department lobby. What could Kevin be doing now? We just discharged him a couple hours ago!

Kevin was a regular, a "frequent flyer." If the emergency department was an airline, he would be played by George Clooney. Kevin visited the emergency department almost every night intoxicated and not farm league intoxicated, but professionally intoxicated – Wheaties box intoxicated. Kevin was a local drunkard who drank himself into homelessness. His alcohol also contributed to a divorce and a myriad of other problems. He was infamous around town. He now spent his time drinking cheap vodka and costing the city and the local hospitals an estimated one million dollars per year.

The emergency department was full – as usual. Tonight most of the patients were actual sick people, which is not always the case. I could not recall a time Kevin had visited with an actual emergency. I doubted tonight was any different.

Susan and I walked down the hallway and through the security door to the lobby. Kevin stood facing the Cat in the Hat statue with his pants around his ankles. The statue was part of the department remodel décor and one of the only Dr. Seuss pieces not in the children's ward. Kevin relieved himself on the statue. Tonight, the trickster cat got more than he bargained for. Kevin showered the Cat with an impressive stream of golden urine. From the looks on the faces on the people in the packed lobby, I do not think they expected a show during their wait. An older couple both looked on mouths agape at the sight of Kevin's antics. The woman did not seem to mind the skin tear on her arm anymore.

"Should I call security?" asked Susan.

No. "Pick up your pants! What are you doing Kevin?" I startled the poor guy and he nearly fell over into the statue when he tried to pull up his pants. He was still peeing and the urine soaked through his dirty khakis and ran down his leg. Everything smelled of cheap vodka. I grabbed his arm and led him back to the department. He nearly fell down when we got to the security door. I held him up when I entered in the door code. He is too drunk to discharge.

"I am sorry," Kevin said looking at me as sincerely as he could. His forehead and scalp were covered in healing scrapes from his numerous visits to the ground. He smelled of body odor, new and old urine – and booze, of course.

"I know you are, Kevin. I know you are."

"Why did you bring him back here? We have no beds yet and he is the last person I would have brought back! There are some actual patients waiting!" yelled Jami, the charge nurse. Jami was mad and stressed. She was always flustered the nights she was the charge nurse. Kevin just gave her somewhere to direct her stress.

"I know, but he was showing his distaste for Dr. Seuss by pissing all over the Cat in the Hat and exposing himself to the lobby. I think he is too drunk to discharge. He cannot ambulate on his own."

"He seems to be walking just fine," said the doctor. The doctor sorted through the stack of charts in the "To be seen" pile and found Kevin's. He quickly filled it out and tossed it into the discharge box. I stood there holding Kevin up.

"We have to call the police Kevin. You are going to have to sleep this off in jail!" Jami told him.

"I am sorry," said Kevin.

The police arrived quickly and took Kevin into custody for the night. The police would either take him to the drunk-tank at the jail or release him down the street. Either way he would be back. He always came back.

Kevin made another appearance two days later. This time, he traveled in style and arrived via ambulance. The ambulance ride gave him gurney service, bypassing the lobby and direct admission to the department. No waiting for Kevin today.

"Kevin was sleeping in the casino again. Weren't you Kevin?" the paramedic asked him and rubbed his sternum. Kevin flinched and growled, but made no other response. He was going to need to sleep this one off for awhile.

"Put him in a hallway bed with the others," Jami ordered the medics. It was another full department night, but this time Kevin had some company. The hall beds were full of intoxicated patients. Using the hallways for patients was frowned upon, but it was a small emergency department and the monitored rooms were needed for people who were really sick. We made do with the resources we had available. I grabbed a portable blood pressure machine and headed toward Kevin to get his vital signs.

"I need to get your temperature Kevin. Open your mouth. We need to see how much alcohol you drank Kevin. Blow on the straw!" Kevin growled and rolled onto his side showing me his back. I used the temporal thermometer to get his temperature and had the doctor order a blood alcohol. Tori, the unlucky nurse assigned to the hallway patients walked over to get a report from the paramedics. She gave the gurney a gentle kick when she approached. "Why did you have to ruin my night Kevin?" she asked infuriated. He growled again. She went about assessing her new patient.

The department was on edge today. It was over capacity and every other patient had a gastrointestinal bleed, so the department smelled like excrement, blood, and vomit. There were also a lot of patients complaining of shortness of breath and chest pain, as well as, the smell of the department. The patients in the hallway were not helping with the smell either. They provided the aroma with a hint of vodka and whiskey. They also took away a limited staff from truly sick patients.

On nights like tonight, the drunken patients really belonged to me. I was responsible for checking on them and maintaining current vital signs until the doctor made time to evaluate them. I knew it would take awhile tonight. The doctor was alone and was on-and-off the phone trying to free up beds by getting patients admitted upstairs. The hospitalist was taking his time coming down stairs to assess patients and we needed beds for people waiting in the lobby. Kevin and the other intoxicated patients' charts remained in the "To be seen" pile.

"Wake up Kevin! We need to talk." I gave him a sternal rub and he growled. I asked again, but he did not respond. I took another blood pressure and it was high as usual. His oxygen saturation was okay. I tried to roll him on his back and he batted my hand away. "I will see you in a bit Kevin." I moved on to the next patient in the hallway. She sat up on the gurney.

"Can I have a sandwich?" she asked.

"I will see what I can do, but first we need to get some vitals." She offered her arm.

Later I made my way back to Kevin. He was still lying on his side. "Kevin! It is time to wake up!" I tapped the gurney rail and shook him by the shoulder. He did not respond. "Kevin?" I rolled him onto his back, gave him a sternal rub, and put the pulse-oximeter on his finger. He still had a pulse and was breathing. I rubbed his sternum again and there was still no response. I picked up his arm and held it above his face and let it fall. He made no effort to stop it and it smacked his face.

"Tori, you need to look at Kevin!" I yelled.

"What is it now?" She asked poking her head out of a patient's room. She tore off a yellow isolation gown and squirted some alcohol into her hands. She put on a new pair of gloves and yelled, "Kevin! Wake up! Kevin!" Dismayed, she grinded her knuckles in his chest.

No response. She lifted his eyelid and paused for a moment. She then shined a pen light across it. No response. His pupils were constricted and non-reactive. "Ah, crap! Get the doctor!"

Everybody had misdiagnosed Kevin this time. He had taken another one of his frequent visits to the ground and landed hard on the back of his head. Kevin was taken to radiology for a CT-scan and we freed up a critical bed for him. The CT-scan confirmed our fears of an intercerebral hemorrhage. The doctor ordered medication intervention to control Kevin's increasing intracranial pressure. Kevin was moved to the intensive care unit later that night and care was transferred to the hospitalists and neurology teams. I think he remained in the hospital for a number of weeks, but you lose track of patients once they leave the emergency department.

"Never make prejudgments about your patients," Dr. Francis said to me. "I think we all forgot that tonight. Luckily we caught the problem soon enough. Good work."

It did not feel like good work. It never did with the homeless drunks. There was little we could do. The treatment programs had waiting lists over a year long, so the social worker could do little. The emergency department was just another rotating door for them. Emergency departments were not designed to be treatment centers for chronic diseases like alcohol dependence.

A physician once told me a joke. It went something like this, "In health care, you need twice the compassion as patience, but without patients you are out of work!" It never was funny and I think it is actually incorrect – having patience is everything in health care. Without patience, your patients will usually disappoint you.

Kevin continued to be a frequent flyer of the emergency department well beyond the day I resigned. I recently read, however, that he has been sober for ten weeks under court order and placed in an experimental recovery program. He has also found employment and is working on his relationship with his estranged wife. Good for him. ☼

Robert Hill is a student at Barry University currently pursuing his dream to becoming a medical doctor.

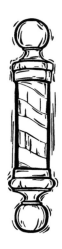

Butchered

By Jacqueline Sanchez

I had been warned by my grandmother and mother, but I suppose I had never fully understood what the warnings meant, or that one human being could actually be so cruel to another. It was a rite of passage, they called it. It was part of our religion, they had told me. No man would want to marry me, they said. In a strange way, I had grown to want it done. So when the day came, I decided to be the brave 7-year-old child I knew everyone else wanted me to be.

I waited in the room all day long, the same room my grandfather had died in that summer, until the time came that my mother ushered in four or five older women, and a man. He was intimidatingly large, with a poorly tucked in shirt, and sweat trickling down his sideburns, and as he came closer, I realized I had seen him before. The man who had trimmed my father's beard so many times, the village barber, was now going to trim me. Before long, I was being faced by him, he who now stood at the edge of the bed between my legs. I lie there, exposed in all the glory I had. He took out a pouch, opened it onto the bed, and made his choice: a straight razor.

I held my breath as he made the first cut. I tried desperately to focus on the ceiling, but the stinging of my sliced flesh prevented me. I struggled to escape, but I couldn't move. Two of the women were holding my legs down, and I was being restrained from behind. I frantically searched the room. I couldn't find my mother.

"Mama," I cried out, wondering where she had gone, why she had abandoned me.

"Hold still, my love," she whispered, "it's ok." I quickly realized she was the one whose arms were wrapped tightly around me. My own mother. How could she let this strange man put his hands on me? Did she know what he was going to do?

"Mama," I pleaded. "It hurts, mama!"

"Cut it! Cut it quickly," one of the women yelled.

As the barber got closer, I could smell stale tobacco on his hot breath, see dirt under his fingernails. I cried harder. Periodically he would lift up, and drop a piece of my womanhood on a nearby table. If this is what it took to be a woman, I didn't want to be one anymore. What was wrong with what I had before? What was wrong with what I had been created with?

I could feel the wetness of my blood under my legs, and the tugging of my lips as they sewed them together with wire. After the man was done, the women brought my legs together, and bound them with cloth, so that my footsteps wouldn't be too far apart to rip the stitches. To them, and to my mother, I was now a woman. A 7-year-old woman, ready to be bought for marriage.

I really was a walking shell, a mere womb. They had made me nothing but a hole that defined my worth as a human being. Sanctified and mutilated, I was now worth nothing but the price a man would one day pay to marry my tightened vagina and my virginity, only to have me for his own consumption, for me to bear his children.

When I was 11, I became very ill. It wasn't until I was taken to a doctor that they realized I had been menstruating, but the blood had had no where to go. So he cut me open, only to sew me back up to a little less than I had originally been, so that I could properly bleed. It was just enough to make the infections go away.

Now at 32, I live with several constant reminders of how my mother and village took away my womanhood that day. Not only will I never experience sexual pleasure, but I will never experience childbirth, as the infections took that from me. I will also never know what it truly is to feel like a woman.

I was very angry for a long time, but I have since forgiven my mother. She knew not that what she had me endure was not indeed a religious obligation, but a morally corrupt and selfish tradition. Countless generations of women before me were butchered and circumcised, and there have been countless after me. I just hope these women one day come to forgive their mothers, and protect their own daughters, allowing them to grow up to be the whole women we were prevented from being. ☼

Jacqueline Sanchez is a graduate student at Barry University.

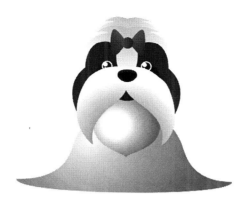

Therapy Dog

By Amy Olivares

The medical chart read: "Margaret Miller, age 9, cerebral palsy." Before I was able to replace the chart back on the door, Nurse Mindy, in her Minnie Mouse scrubs, stopped dead in her tracks as if a red light had caught her by surprise. She looked at Dr. Gracie, gave her a pat on the head and said, "She needs to see you stat!"

You see, Dr. Gracie is not a pediatric surgeon or a nurse. Dr. Gracie's hospital name-badge reads:

Dr. Gracie
Pediatrics Chief Resident
K-9 unit

Gracie is part of a special group of therapy dogs that visit the children in the pediatrics wing of Miami Children's Hospital. Standing only nine inches tall and weighing in at a mere fifteen pounds, Gracie is a happy, healthy, high-spirited eight-year-old Shih Tzu. She knows what her purpose is once her paws cross the sliding glass doors labeled "Authorized Personnel Only." Once she is through those portals, she is no longer just a pet, she is a therapist.

I returned the chart back to its holder, looked down at Gracie and said, "Are you ready?" Her ears perked up as she looked at me with her charcoal eyes, and with a single wag of her tail, walked into Margaret's room.

The walls were plastered with cartoons that seemed to come alive. Through the single window in the room you could see the hospital playground.

Off in the corner of the room sat Margaret's father, with his face burrowed in his hands. He cried. I whispered, "This is Gracie, and she is here to see Margaret." He slowly raised his face from his hands and nodded his approval.

With a disheartened look at Gracie, he said, "Margaret has not moved or said a word in weeks. She has limited mobility and is barely responsive."

With one look at Margaret, I thought this might be a bad idea. Gracie was used to children who would pet her and let her give them lady-like but wet, sloppy kisses. She had never interacted with a child in this condition.

I decided that Gracie could handle this. I asked, "Is it okay if I place Gracie on the bed?"

"Sure," he said with a feeble shrug.

I placed Gracie at the foot of the bed, something I had done many times before; however, this time it was different. Gracie did not quickly run up to Margaret and beg for belly rubs as she usually did. This time she crawled towards Margaret's immobile hand, maneuvering through all the medical IVs like a combat soldier in a mine field.

Gracie lay next to Margaret for a few moments. She nuzzled her wet nose up against Margaret's middle finger and gave it a soft lick. Margaret, ever so slightly, raised her finger. Taking that as an invitation, Gracie inched over the polka-dotted bed sheets and laid nose-to-nose with Margaret. With her big eyes, she looked in Margaret's gaze and licked her nose. Even though Gracie just lay next to Margaret for a few minutes, it seemed as if they were best friends. Right before I lifted Gracie off the bed, I said, "Goodbye." Gracie gave Margaret another lick and to this Margaret let out a barely audible giggle and smiled.

Margaret's father diverted his gaze from Gracie to Margaret and then back to Gracie. As I re-hooked Gracie's leash onto her hospital pet therapy vest and exited the room, Margaret's father smiled and said, "Thanks."

Gracie and I continued to visit children. She let anyone and everyone give her a belly rub. In return she would give a wet and sloppy kiss. She, of course, was not picky or selective about whom she kissed. The more the merrier.

The next week, when Gracie and I returned, Nurse Mindy handed me an envelope and walked off.

Two words were written on the envelope: "To Gracie." I found a nearby bench and sat down. I opened the envelope and found a letter from Margaret's father:

Dear Gracie,

Margaret passed away shortly after your visit. She died in her sleep. I will truly miss my baby girl. I want to thank you for giving me the best final gift a parent could ask for. I saw my child smile one last time. That is how I will remember Margaret, with you by her side with that smile on her face. Thank you.

Sincerely,
Sam Miller, Margaret's Dad

I paused to think about what I had just read and looked down at Gracie who sat patiently by my side.

Gracie as always, looked up at me with her big dark eyes as if to say, "We need to see patients." ☀

Amy Olivares is a student at Barry University working on her Masters Degree in Biomedical Sciences.

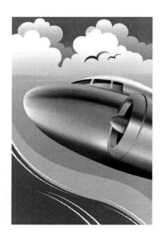

The Plane Truth

By Mort Laitner

I picked up the letter, observed the return address was that of a Circuit Court Judge, and tore into it. As I ripped the envelope, it reminded me of the horrifying feeling of getting grades in the mail. I scanned the note, seeing that typed in all caps was the word CONFIDENTIAL and it was signed by the judge. It read:

"I appreciated your response to the request for information.

I will maintain the confidentiality of the information, and appreciate that the involuntary hospitalization only took one day in the United States.

Thank you for your attention to these matters."

So this note would be my reward. With relief, I plunged into my office chair, as if I received that passing grade, smiling and saying, "Thank you Martin Buber for your I and Thou essay. It worked."

I closed my eyes and went back in time---two months, remembering that I sat in this same chair when the phone rang. I picked up the receiver to hear Anthony's familiar voice. The CDC representative said, "Houston, we have a problem. A flight attendant is arriving in an hour at MIA from Spain. She's got active TB---contagious. She absconded from a Madrid hospital against medical advice. She is masked on the plane and no one is seated near her. We would like your assistance in quarantining her."

I replied, "Tony, my friend, I'll jump in my car and I'll be there in thirty minutes. Thanks for the heads up. She sure is breaking the flight attendant's code of being on the plane for the safety and comfort of the passengers. I doubt she is inspiring the confidence of those unlucky stiffs sitting on that jet."

Tony let out a stifled laughed and a curt, "Good-bye."

As questions ran through my head, I pulled out my statute book and quickly read the tuberculosis law. Was this lady a threat to the public health? Was she taking any TB meds? Did she really have this deadly disease? Would the airport provide me with a mask so I could interview her?

I drove to the airport, remembering the stewardesses of the 1950's and 60's. They looked like models, young and shapely in their tightly-fitted uniforms. They wore those cute air hostess hats and for male travelers they were a fringe benefit of flying. These unwed women dressed in their short skirts serving alcohol and dispensing free mini packs of cigarettes were a sight for sore eyes. They were celebrities in an occupation where height and weight limits were as tightly controlled as the cost of a plane ticket. The airlines competed for customers by feeding them steak, mini-lobster tails and this bevy of beauties. I thought, "Boy, times have changed," as I wondered what this attendant would look like.

Walking through the airport, I thought about the requirements I'd have to meet to get the judge to issue an emergency hold on this lady. What would I ask her? What medical records would the CDC have?

Pausing next to the airport hotel entrance, it hit me, EUREKA! —Martin Buber's "I-Thou and I-It relationships."

Here was my chance to conduct a philosophical experiment. I would have a dialogue with this human in need of help. I would treat her not as an object. There would be a dialogue between us, not a monologue. She would listen and be taught about this disease---its risks to her and her family, how the medication worked and what steps she would have to take. She would respond to the experiment by voluntarily agreeing to being examined, tested and hospitalized. There would be no need for the drama of the courtroom.

Arriving at the airport's quarantine station, I met the assembled team: a doctor, some airline personnel and Tony. We discussed the case.

Tony: "The Spanish authorities have emailed us this definitive proof that she has TB. She admitted to it in the Madrid Hospital."

The Doctor: "We will need to have these notes translated into English."

Airline Rep: "You know she stole her medical records from the hospital last night and she got on the plane after her doctors told her not to."

Me to myself: "Maybe this is not the right case to try Buber?"

Then we donned our N-95 masks and proceeded to enter the small bare-walled interviewing room where the flight attendant, "Doris" sat. She was a bit over weight, well-coifed and groomed. But in her uniform she did not reach the standards of those hot steward-esses of my youth. I listened as she denied every material fact—ex-cept, she did admit taking her original medical records from the hospital without their permission. While waiting for the others to complete their questions, I decided to look her in the eyes and try to get the truth out of her. I would attempt to engage her in dialogue, without any qualifications or objectifications---even with the mask on, and it sort of worked.

Doris agreed to go to the health department and the hospital for testing, examination and quarantine without a court order. I didn't believe a word she said. I did not trust her. Doris would run from the hospital the minute we turned our backs. This was not the concrete encounter I envisioned but rather a judgmental cross-examination.

As we waited in the TB clinic for x-rays and other test results, I realized that Doris had not eaten since leaving the plane. I would be treating her as an object (I-It) if I did not order her a meal. She seemed genuinely surprised as I handed her salad and a drink that she had not requested.

While Doris ate and I waited, a health department legal team obtained a hospitalization order to hold her for the next 24 hours. They also hired an armed guard to stop her from escaping.

As night fell upon Jackson Memorial Hospital, getting Doris a bed turned into a nightmare. After waiting two hours for admission, only the threat of reaching top hospital officials rendered any success. I realized how awful the I-It felt.

Before Doris entered her private room, I had the unsavory task of showing and telling her about the 24-hour quarantine order and the armed guard posted outside her room. Now Doris realized I did not trust her and she flipped out. I had seen her Dr. Jekyll, and now I witnessed her Mr. Hyde. Remaining calm and listening paid off, as finally Doris accepted her fate and the short-story book I gave her. A tired Doris called it a night.

The next morning Doris and the team learned her TB tests came back negative. She had told some truth and she was allowed to fly home. I had already apologized to her the night before just in case she was free of TB but explained we had a job to do in protecting the public's health.

A month later Doris wrote the judge who signed the quarantine order asking for some blood---specifically mine. The judge issued an order requesting information as to what happened.

Again I thought Martin Buber and in my I-Thou response, I spoke of our team effort, the information received from Spain and the stolen medical records. My heart-felt story and the judge's kind and appreciative response created that dialogue I wanted.

Eureka the experiment worked! ☼

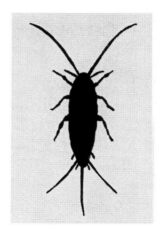

Cooties

By Linda Ying

"Hey, sis. Can you take me to the hospital?"

My pen paused in the middle of my precise note-taking, and I peered suspiciously at my brother leaning casually in my doorway. "And…" I replied with exaggerated slowness, "dare I ask exactly why you so urgently need to go to the hospital?"

He dropped his eyes from my piercing gaze, and began shuffling his feet across my carpeted floor. "Well, you see… The thing is…" He began wringing his hands so violently that it left bright red marks on his pale skin. "I just found out that…" he trailed off in a low voice, all the while still not lifting his face to meet my stare. I was beginning to get a little angry. I had no time to play games. I had notes to rewrite, a two-hour lecture to listen to, and 60 plus pages of biology to read. But as I opened my mouth to yell, I remembered with sudden clarity the secret he revealed and begged me not to tell our parents. I even remember how he had started the conversation with a casual, "So, what do you think if I got myself a girlfriend…"

"Oh my god," I moaned, my eyes widening in shock. "You caught something from her, didn't you? Or, or… oh no, did you get her pregnant?" I rose quickly to my feet, not caring that my thigh struck the desk with enough force to send my notes fluttering to the ground. It was only later that I noticed the blackish-purple bruise shaped like a kidney on my upper leg.

His own eyes bulged out of their sockets, as if he did not have enough air, and his mouth dropped in a comical "O" of surprise. His complexion, usually fair, reddened until it seemed like he had spent hours outside in the burning sun. "No!!" He screamed in a high pitched voice that only dogs could hear. "That's not it at all! Besides, we haven't even…" He choked off the last few words, blushing even more furiously, and started twisting his hands into irregular shapes again.

I sank slowly back unto my seat, breathing a deep sigh of relief. I felt like I had just barely escaped with my life by jumping out from the front of a speeding train at the last second. "So if that's not it, then why?" I inquired, full of curiosity.

"Well, she's been feeling sick lately, and yesterday…" He took a deep breath and babbled out without pausing, "shefoundoutthatshe-hasmonoandIneedtogettested." As he stood there shame-faced like a little boy that had stolen out of the cookie jar, I attempted to process the information I had been given. So I said the first thing that popped into my head. "What's mono?"

"You know, mono." He gestured dramatically with his hands in the air. I responded with a steady blank stare. "It's also called the Kissing Disease."

"Oh, so you basically got cooties from her?" I blurted out without thinking. His fury was immediate, and I cowered like the sailors did in the face of Poseidon's anger. "Can you please just take me to the hospital?"

And so I shut my mouth and played the role of the older, protective sister. I was able to find a clinic that could squeeze us in the very same day. As he sat in the empty waiting room with the neon green clipboard balanced on his knobby knees, filling out his medical information, I was already hatching schemes on how to quarantine him.

As I was mentally ticking off items I would have to purchase at the grocery store, a soft voice interrupted, calling my brother's name. The time had come. It was his turn to finally find out if he was infected. Before the door closed behind him, he glanced back anxiously. I gave him a thumbs-up, and my goofiest grin, hoping to encourage him a little. The door swung shut, and I was left alone to stare at the graphic posters decorating the walls that warned irresponsible adults to get tested for various STD's. The seconds ticked into long minutes, and I felt like I was in court awaiting the jury for a verdict.

Finally, I heard the soft squeak of the door opening, and I looked up to see my brother coming out, with a dazed look on his face. "I don't have it, " he said slowly, gazing stupidly at me. "I don't have mono."

I clapped him smartly on the back, steered him toward the door, and began guiding him out to the brightly shining sun. "Great! Now I don't have to kick you out of the apartment."

To this day, he still has no idea how he dodged the bullet, even though he shared practically everything with his girlfriend. I always tell him not to worry about it, and to just feel lucky he didn't get sick. And I can never help poking fun of him by singing, "Circle, circle, dot, dot, now you've got the cootie shot!"

Linda Ying is a student in the Biomedical Sciences Masters program at Barry University in Miami Shores, Florida.

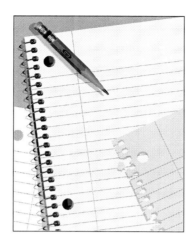

The Note

By Mort Laitner

I yanked open my top desk drawer searching for an old piece of paper—a folded, yellowish note pad page. Scrawled across that page, I had written a message to myself. The note traveled with me from Miami to St. Pete, to Baton Rouge and back to Miami. It lived in at least six different desks over the past forty years. The note and I traveled from school to school, and from job to job. I'd clear out my old desk, throw the note and all the drawer's contents in a manila envelope, and then dump them in my new desk. The note remained a silent, often ignored companion—a distant reminder of a long unfulfilled goal.

To no avail, I rescanned all my desk drawers while wondering what had happened to it. My luck and the note had gone south. I lost it.

The night before my unsuccessful search, I taught ethics at Barry University. We discussed Kohlberg's Theory of Cognitive Development.

I asked the class, "What other hierarchies have you studied?"

"Maslow's Hierarchy of Needs in Psychology," Hugo replied.

Hugo's words transported me back to 1968—my psychology class at the University of Miami. I scoured the classroom for that cute, buxom, five-foot-three-inch blond. No luck. She usually sat in front of me. Not seeing her, I realized that I did not know her name but had her dimensions branded in my brain. I doubted if she even knew I existed. I lacked the fortitude to introduce myself. My fear of rejection and/or ridicule paralyzed my tongue and lips. I knew I was not fully developed.

I turned my head and my attention to my psych professor as he called the class to order. "Today we are going to study Maslow's Hierarchy of Needs."

I started to take notes as he drew a triangle on the blackboard. He divided the triangle into five sections, with the words "Being Needs" above it and the words "Deficit Needs" below it. As the professor filled in each section, I wondered where I stood on this Hierarchy of Needs.

On a yellowish piece of note paper, I copied the pyramid-shaped list.

Self-actualization

Esteem needs—**Lower**: status, fame, glory, recognition. **Higher**: self-respect, confidence, understanding, goodness, justice, beauty, order, and symmetry.

Love and Belongingness needs—affiliation, acceptance, affection.

Safety needs—job security, financial reserves, living in safe environment.

Physiological needs—air, food, water, sleep, sex.

The cute blond arrived, took her seat, and whipped out her spiral pad. As she copied the list, I pondered where she fit in this hierarchy. I guessed she rested a notch or two higher than me.

When the class ended, I took one last long look at the blond as she exited the room. I folded Maslow's list and carefully placed it in my wallet. I decided that I would examine the note annually to determine if I had met my new goal of self-actualization.

I snapped back to teaching and asked my student Hugo, "What did Maslow consider the ultimate stage a person could attain in his hierarchy?"

"Self-actualization," Hugo replied.

"And what is self-actualization?" I queried.

"Professor, it's the summit, the apex, the top. It's when one reaches his or her full potential as a person. However the person's needs are never fully satisfied because there are always new opportunities for continued growth."

Massaging my chin, I replied, "Hugo, I'm quite impressed with your memory. Do you have any more info on this subject?"

"Professor, I do. The self-actualized have a sense of humility and a deep respect for others. They are compassionate and have strong ethics. They are creative, problem solving folks with a sense of humor that is not hostile. The self-actualized have frequent peak experiences, by which I mean, moments of profound happiness or harmony. Existence on this planet being so tough, I'm not surprised that only a small percentage of people are self-actualized—Maslow thinks around two percent. In fact, I'm not sure I know or have met any of them."

I addressed the class, "Are any of you self-actualized?"

No hands went up, and silence enveloped the room.

I felt the students' eyes rest upon me. They looked curiously at me as a smile broke across my face. In a moment of clarity, I realized I had met my goal. I had made it!

It took forty years, but the note had burned a mental road map for my self development. I had just tasted another profound moment of happiness and harmony. I let out a muffled laugh as I wondered whatever happened to the cute blonde. ☼

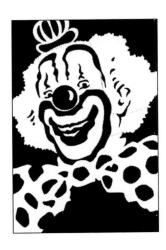

Rest in Peace

By Mort Laitner

I sat in McDonald's drinking my senior-priced coffee and eating my fruit and maple oatmeal. I loved the taste of the multiple flavors blending in my mouth. I cherished the smell of the coffee wafting through my nostrils. I smiled and thought it's good to eat healthy and cheap. My breakfast consisted of 32 grams of natural Quaker oats, with soluble and insoluble fiber, (the fiber maintains blood sugar control by slowing down food digestion) cream, brown sugar and a half a cup of diced apples, cranberries and raisins equaling 290 calories. If I asked for no sugar it would have been 260.

With the corner of my eye I glanced at the eatery's entrance and observed an obese male speeding in his electric-powered wheelchair toward the front door. His face covered in beads of sweat. A bulbous red-veined nose yelled about years of over consumption of alcohol. His fiery eyes danced in his head. In his right hand his pudgy fingers held an 8 1/2 by 11 inch white piece of paper and in his left a long piece of scotch-tape. Here was a man on a mission, with a message I had to read.

I watched as he taped his missive to the door. Then the fat man sped away. I ran to the door to read and retrieved the note, knowing full well how quickly the store's employees would tear it down and throw it in the trash.

As I sipped my coffee I read:

R.I.P.

Ronald McDonald

1963-2011

I will miss you my skinny curly red-headed friend.

Your smile is known around the world.

You were our clown, our joy, our laughter. You put happy in the toy-laden Happy Meal. Your face adorned that colorful box which we read as we munched out on your burgers and those animal cracker cookies.

Boy did you make us laugh in your commercials, cartoons, and video games. Your picture was plastered throughout the store. I remember those thirty-second commercials of you and your friends, Mayor McCheese, Hamburglar and Grimace bombarding the airwaves every Saturday morning. We were there with you in McDonaldland. I recall seeing statues of you sitting on a bench, standing and waving to your fans sprouted up in all the stores' playgrounds. With the grand-opening of a new store, you would make a personal appearance and we clamored to shake your hand.

I remember as a ten year-old, my friends and I begged our parents to drive thirty miles from Woodridge to Middletown for one of your 15 cent burgers. In the family Ford Fairlane we headed south toward those Golden Arches and dreamed of those oil drenched, steaming hot salt-covered fries housed in their white paper holder. Those hot fries melted on contact with the interior of your mouth as they travelled to your gut. Our taste buds relished this overdose of salt. Then we cooled our mouths with ice cold coke.

As I travelled the globe you were there. I remembered the religious experience of seeing the sun careening off of the Golden Arches as I drove over the hills surrounding Jerusalem and wondering if Ronald wore a kippa.

You brought joy to millions of kids around the world by wearing that red and white striped long-sleeved shirt with your yellow vest and gloves. We bought billions of your burgers in your honor.

Your doll rested on my children's bed for years. We loved buying your coke-filled glasses. Those brightly colored drinking glasses, with your picture plastered on all sides, adorned our kitchen until they broke from overuse.

How many times did I visit the store as a child, as a high school and college student, as a parent/grandparent? At least twice a week—times fifty-two weeks times fifty years for a grand total of five thousand two hundred visits to McDonalds.

Good-bye my skinny, curly red-headed friend.

Rest in peace Ronald.

I will miss you.

I scanned the restaurant for images of this icon. There were none to be found. Where was he hiding? Why was he absent? Who would fill those big red shoes? Could this be the result of the fast food chain being accused of making American children obese? Was Ronald on his way to become the poster boy for obesity?

As I approached the counter for a refill I looked down at the nation's, tzedakah (charity) box. I observed the box loaded with coins and paper currency, realizing the beauty of America's religious obsession with giving to Ronald McDonald House. Here we were following one of Rambam's highest levels of giving to charity. On the box, I saw the last vestige of Ronald in the store, a half-inch house, with the insignia for Ronald McDonald Foundation. The foundation that provides homes away from home for children and their relatives when a child is hospitalized—with their moving slogan, "Keeping families together when they need it most." In their logo, there were two shaking hands, one was clearly Ronald's, yellow gloved with the golden arch and a red-and-white striped sleeve, while the other hand represented the contributing public.

I thought of the eulogy-posting, wheelchair man's pudgy fingers grasping Ronald's hand for one last shake as he whispered "Ronald, thanks for all the memories."

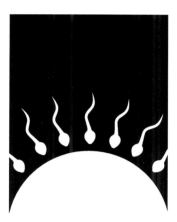

Nine Months in Hell

By Kimberly Lamothe

When I first found out I was pregnant, I was just as stupefied as most women. After all, I had been training to take care of a baby since I was a little girl, playing with my dolls and treating them like newborns. The only difference was that I never played "being pregnant," and I definitely never played "being pregnant with Hyperemesis Gravidorum." Never was I told that morning sickness lasts all day, or that the smell or the sight of certain things, including my husband, would make me vomit. I had always imagined the baby-carrying process consisting of getting fat and nine months later screaming for two Hollywood minutes to give birth to a precious baby doll in a hospital room surrounded by loved ones. Well, my pregnancy was anything but the traditional gestation.

Three months into my pregnancy, having lost 20 pounds, I was feeling like this was not what I had signed up for, this was not what happened when the princesses from my fairytales married their Prince Charmings and had babies. The fairytale princesses did not have Hyperemesis Gravidorum. As a matter of fact, the average woman does not know about Hyperemesis Gravidorum either. Only a lucky 1% of us suffer from HG, and I blamed my mother. Scientists have only been able to attribute this terrible condition to genetic predisposition. HG is nothing like the average morning sickness that women experience during their first trimester. The average HG sufferer vomits at least 10 times a day and loses anywhere from 5 to 30% of her body weight. This drastic weight loss is of course accompanied by dehydration. To add insult to injury, the antiemetics used in chemotherapy prescribed to HG women also carry severe constipation as a side effect. An HG woman is fortunate if she has a bowel movement once a week.

I went from being a student and a worker to a gravid couch potato, except instead of expanding and eating cupcakes and ding-dongs like most pregnant women, I was shrinking more and more every day. By the end of my pregnancy catastrophe, I was 40 lbs lighter and 10 lbs away from anorexia. With my gravid belly, I looked like an adult with kwashiorkor syndrome, which is a disease prominent among children in third world countries like Haiti. My dehydrated skin resembled that of an African lizard. While most pregnant women are busy keeping a journal throughout their pregnancy, I was figuring out what I could eat for dinner that would be less painful as it traveled back up my esophagus accompanied by the burning sensation of my acidic gastric secretions. In the mornings, my husband was greeted by my bright yellow bile in the white bucket smelling like a mixture of rotten eggs and hot dogs.

The baby books say to read, talk, and even sing to the baby within the womb, but I was too bitter. I had nothing good to say. It felt as if an alien was growing in my stomach, sucking out all of my life and energy, and whatever was left of me was in the bucket by my bed waiting for my husband to clean it up when he came home from work every night.

Difficult as it was to endure physically and emotionally, I wish I had thought of my unborn baby as a blessing like most women. I compare my HG suffering to that of a person suffering from cancer. There is of course, a major difference: at end of the long catastrophic venture, I was free of all sickness and blessed with a smaller than average but nonetheless beautiful munchkin. ✺

Kimberly Lamothe is a graduate student at Barry University in Miami Shores and an aspiring gynecologist. However, she insists that her most treasured and rewarding jobs are to be a mother to 10 month old Gabriel and a loving wife to Greg. Kimberly and Greg plan on having more children despite her childbearing struggles.

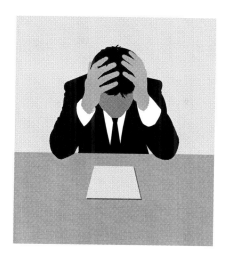

Over and Over and Over Again

By Anonymous

I sit on the floor of my apartment crying. The soft carpet beneath me and the only thing I see above me is the ceiling. I can't move. I don't want to move. I know that moving would just make everything more difficult. My mind keeps drifting back from the thought of walking through the door to the thought of me getting up from the floor. Everything is difficult right now and it seems to happen so quickly. I keep thinking, "How did I end up like this?"

When I was fourteen, the first symptoms of my Obsessive-Compulsive Disorder (OCD) started showing up. I remember when washing my hands I would lather, rinse, and repeat in multiples of four. Most of the time I would end up washing them until my hands were raw. I didn't care, at least I felt good about it. At the time I didn't understand why it made me feel better, but I simply accepted it for what it was.

When I was seventeen, the theme of my OCD changed. I still washed my hands in multiples of four, but the OCD had become more of a mind game. I felt it necessary to think about someone I respected, my father, while doing some things, such as getting in and out of bed or walking through a doorway. If when doing these things I happened to think about someone I didn't respect, the President at the time, I found myself having to repeat the action over and over again until I only thought about my father. Now it might seem easy to do this, but try not thinking about something. For example, don't think about a pink elephant. What are you thinking about? I bet it's a pink elephant.

My life seemed to end when I entered college. My OCD became worse and eventually it was all-consuming. I reached a point in my life where I couldn't do much of anything. Every time I wanted to do something I realized that in order for me to do it right I had to obey the illogical laws of my OCD. It took me a minimum of two grueling hours to get to class. I started missing classes because I couldn't seem to get anywhere in time. At a certain point I became so fed up with it and so depressed because of it that I rarely left the house. I soon realized that I was too afraid to do anything--too fearful to face what lie ahead.

The depression and fear of moving took over. I spiraled down-ward. The only reason I woke up every morning was because I didn't really have a choice in the matter. I became a recluse. I never left my bed. I only got up to eat and stay hygienic, which took me several hours, so I had a pretty busy day. My grades started falling and I reached a state at which I had to make a choice whether to stay in bed for the rest of my life or to do something about my little problem. Medication and therapy is just what the doctor ordered.

Two years passed. It was two years filled with different kinds of pills and hours of insightful talking. At the end of it all I found a medication that helped make things a little better and I came to an important conclusion. I was never going to be completely cured because there was no cure. This was something I had to live with and accept. Throughout my entire experience with OCD so far the hardest part has been accepting it.

Today I have come a long way since that time in my life when I was scared to leave the bed. My grades improved. I'm taking steps to pursue a career in medicine and eventually plan on helping others like me. Doing even the simplest tasks is more difficult than necessary, but I've learned a few techniques to make it a little easier. But more importantly, I've learned how to make it through the day.

Thinking back to the path I took with my OCD makes it a little easier to get up from the floor and face what's ahead. I take a deep breath and complete the most difficult step: standing up. Slowly but surely I make my way to the door and step out. I stare at the door and take a minute to think about everything again. I think about the different phases I went through. I think about the range of emotions I went through: periods of depression, anger, denial, bargaining, and acceptance. I even think about how difficult this is going to be. Thinking about accepting it all makes this whole ordeal seem easier though, even if it isn't any different from every other time I've tried to walk through a door.

I step through the door carefully thinking about three people that I respect while trying not to think about anyone else. The first try, I get it wrong. Second try, wrong. Third try, again I get it wrong. Each time I get it wrong I step back outside. I take a deep breath and step through the door. Finally I get it right. I take out my phone and look at pictures of the people I was thinking about and listen to a voice recording of each of their voices saying "I love you." If I didn't do that I know that I would've seen pictures of the people I don't respect and would have to repeat everything over. This is just in case.

Finally I reach the couch, sit down and eat lunch. This all was so that I could eat lunch.

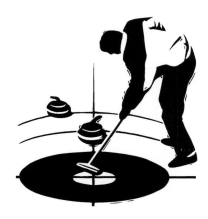

Swept Up

By Amy Tejirian

"Harder! Harder!" a slim, athletic woman shouted. I was mesmerized by what I was watching on television. I sat on the edge of my chair in anticipation. Two other women clad in identical attire ran across the screen sweeping vigorously with brooms in hand. A large, red stone glided until it hit a yellow stone with such force that both shot in opposite directions.

"Yeah!" I exclaimed as if the athletes could hear me. It was 2006 and I was watching curling at the XX Winter Olympic Games in Torino, Italy.

What is curling? Many think of lifting weights or curling hair when I mentioned the name of the sport.

In brief, curling is of Scottish origin and is similar to shuffle board or bocce ball but is played on ice. Four players on each team take turns to slide eight forty-two-pound rocks of granite across the ice into a bulls-eye called the house. Whichever team lands their stone closer to the bulls-eye wins. They get a point for each stone they have in the house that is closer than the first closest stone of their opponent. One round is called an end. In the Olympics, ten ends are considered a match.

Why do they sweep? Teammates sweep rocks for two reasons. The rock's natural inclination is to curl down the ice. Sweeping in front of it makes it travel straight. Also, sweeping makes the stone go a little further.

Curling is a sport that requires much strategy and is sometimes referred to as chess on ice.

My interest in curling began when I was a little girl learning about the Winter Olympics in school in preparation for the XV games that were coming to my hometown, Calgary, Alberta, Canada. It looked like fun. The 1988 games were the first time since 1932 that curling would be an exhibition sport. It finally became a contested sport with medals ten years later in Nagano, Japan.

After watching the 2006 games, I wanted to learn to curl. I was tired of being a sedentary observer. I wanted to get out and experience throwing a stone, sweeping the ice, and cheering my teammates. This was one Olympic sport that looked like any ordinary person, such as myself, could play unlike other sports, like ski jumping. However, living in South Florida made it an obstacle. I posted a question online as to where the closest curling rink was. A couple of people replied with comments like, "In Florida? Good luck." One person was surprised that someone in South Florida would even know what curling was. I was dismayed at learning to curl any time soon or as long as I lived in a tropical region.

As the 2010 Olympics approached, I got antsy to watch the sport again on television and live vicariously through the athletes. One day as I was sitting at a Florida Panthers game during intermission, something on the jumbotron caught my eye. It read "Want to learn how to curl?"

Was I reading this right? Did it just ask what I thought, what I hoped, it had asked? I took a second glance and just stared at the screen in awe. Then I quickly jumped up, grabbed the phone from my purse and dialed the number displayed on the jumbotron. I placed the phone under my ear but couldn't hear anything so I ran to the lobby. I think someone answered when the ringing stopped but she was barely audible.

"I want to learn to curl!" I shouted.

"What?" the lady replied.

I repeated myself but so did the lady. I gave up, tried to say goodbye and returned to my seat vowing that I would call the number tomorrow.

The next day I learned that there would be curling lessons in the winter.

Finally, I was at the "Learn to Curl" event. I anticipated this moment for so long, I didn't know what to expect. We first watched a movie that explained the game, its rules and lingo. Then, the moment had arrived. Each participant wore a "slider" shoe cover on one foot and a "gripper" shoe cover on the other. We first learned to properly move on the ice with these. Then we started to throw the heavy stones. Everyone fell that day, except the instructors. But by the end of the session, we had gotten the grasp of the game. We even played an end or two. Everyone was having so much fun that we forgot about the time and played until two in the morning. Then, as customary, we all gathered at the bar for a beer and to socialize. What an awesome game!

After the first time I curled, I was swept up in the fun. I tried to attend as many Learn to Curl events as I could but they were all full due to the sudden popularity of the sport. The 2010 Winter Olympics in Vancouver had just started, and NBC was airing a lot of the curling matches. They even cracked a joke that NBC stood for Nothing But Curling.

A few instructors were talking about starting a curling league. Of course I would join. So now every Wednesday night for the last two years, I drive over 50 miles to go curl with the new Panthers Curling Club.

Although I curl to have fun, it is also beneficial for the body. To stay healthy, the Centers for Disease Control and Prevention recommends that adults get at least a hundred and fifty minutes of physical activity each week. Going to a gym and using a stationary machine is boring to me. Instead of viewing it as a chore, I'd rather enjoy myself like doing a hobby. Curling is the perfect outlet to keep physically fit. I don't even realize that I am exercising, but after two hours of play, I burn over four hundred calories.

Curling is an anaerobic sport as most players must sweep briskly up and down the ice then calm down enough to throw the rock. Strength in the core is needed to sustain quality sweeping. Leg-muscle strength is also important for curlers to maintain the stone delivery position for any length of time because the quadriceps carry most of the body weight during the slide.

I not only get a great workout, but I have also made great friends. Other unique and unexpected surprises have occurred. I appeared on television curling in a commercial on Fox Sports. Most memorable is that I actually got to meet and curl with Jason Smith, one of the athletes for the USA that I watched on TV during the Vancouver Olympics. I'm no longer just a spectator but I an avid participant.

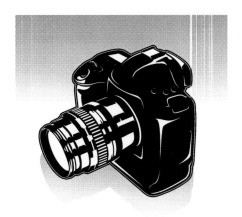

Take a Friggin Picture

By Patrick Lewis

B OOM, SCREECH, ERRRR. These three sounds were the only sounds to describe what just happened. The word "crap" comes to mind, as to the extent in which this young boy's life just changed.

Picture a five year-old boy with nothing but a bright, skies-the-limit-future ahead of him. While skateboarding, he did notice, a "ginormous" Ford Bronco that would make this day, the last one he would ever ride that skateboard. His body was taken like a set of clothes in a dryer, being spun three-hundred-sixty degrees going through multiple rotations with the tire of the Ford Bronco. He tossed like a rag doll, before the truck could come to a complete stop.

One day he was considered a "normal" child, whatever normal is considered at the age of five, and then a life defining moment changed it all. Unfortunately, or fortunately, depending who you are, this boy had no say that his life-defining moment just occurred in the blink of an eye.

At the time, skateboarding was the popular activity in the neighborhood. Having just been given a new skateboard the week before, it was an all day activity for this particular boy. He would get up early and practice daily. However, living on a hill, his favorite part of having his own skateboard was sitting on the skateboard and riding down the hill to the parallel neighbor's driveway.

No longer allowed to grow up like a five year-old should, he was on the brink of death. Doctors diagnosed him with a trauma-induced stroke, leaving him with an incurable muscle disorder referred to as dystonia, a disorder that causes excessive muscle contractions throughout his left side, uncontrollable muscle spasms, and all-day discomfort that most will never have to feel for a minute of their lives.

Over the years, growing up was different for him than most. Most children are able to start playing little league sports at the age of eight or nine, but for him sports were merely a spectator experience until he was eleven. Not able to play baseball, basketball or soccer with his friends, he had to watch his younger brother enjoy all the fun of athletics. He did not think it was fair. Instead of playing hours of sports, he had to go through hours of rehab each week, missing out on special events at school due to physical and occupational therapy.

However, missing sports or being left out of school events was not the toughest part for him to overcome. It was the expectations of society. The word normal was used early. Apparently this boy was no longer normal and everyone let him know that by the stares and weird looks at the way he limped or the way he had no control of his left arm. Children, adults, and everyone else stared. He had to work extra hard to fit in, feeling the need to have a close circle of friends that accepted him, in order to overcome the feeling of being different.

As we fast-forward two decades, with years of rehab, countless hours of surgery, the stares still have not stopped. Now, at twenty-six, this man has learned the glaring looks are part of him. Over the years, he has used those looks and doubts as motivation to be the best possible person. Not once does the thought "what if" cross his mind anymore. He knows that his life-defining moment happened when he was five. That moment built him into the strong, dedicated, and confident man he is today.

People think he is disadvantaged in every way. Some think because he had a brain injury, he is not smart. Others think, because he lacks some physical capabilities, that he cannot function as a person. He was and still is the last picked for dodge ball.

Nothing mentioned in this story makes him regret what happened. He not only knows that it made him stronger than everyone that has ever doubted him but has given him a different view on life, that some will never be able to appreciate. He knows he gets benefits beyond belief and gets better parking than most celebrities.

Although he still receives weird looks from people that do not realize everyone is not the same, he now has the confidence to know he is better off. He can look back at those people and say, "Take a friggin picture, it will last longer!" ☀

Patrick Lewis is a student in the Biomedical Sciences Masters program at Barry University in Miami Shores, Florida.

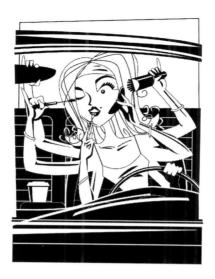

"Oopsies"

By Michelle LeBlanc

L ike a pop star on tour, I rock my head back and forth while I crank up the volume to the song with my favorite lyrics:

"Don't worry about the future; or worry, but know that worrying is as effective as trying to solve an algebra equation by chewing bubblegum. The real troubles in your life are apt to be things that never crossed your worried mind. Don't stress about the small things, the things you should worry about will just hit you."*

Speeding down the highway, top down and wind in my hair, I am lost in my mobile dance party as the Florida sun glistens over my suntan. "Pure ecstasy."

Barely audible over my music, I hear the low but familiar "PING." Robotically my hand searches for my iPhone. I rummage through nail polish bottles, lint removers, hairbrushes, and perfume bottles in search of my ringing phone. After a quick sprtiz of Eau d'Hermes, I forego my search now otherwise distracted by my Kiss-Me-Kate lip gloss. I pull down the vanity mirror, lips shimmering, and check to see that my orange, bug eyed-sunglasses rest perfectly in place. My glasses, combined with my matching orange nails reflect the mood I portray to the world, electrifying and exhilarating. Slurping my fat-free frappichino balanced strategically on my lap, my song ends. I begin a balancing act as my orange blur of fingers punch the pre-set buttons on my stereo.

I suddenly realize I'm missing my turn and exclaim, "Oopsies!" I grab the wheel with both hands, and fling my red Mini Cooper through the intersection and floor the pedal like a NASCAR driver. I hear the screeching of tires and my radio is drowned out by the sound of oncoming horns.

Everything goes black. My car spins uncontrollably and my heart drops to the bottom of my stomach as I feel the twisting of leather as my hands clench the steering wheel.

The muffled sound of sirens brings me to consciousness for a brief moment. I catch a glimpse of shards of glass and metal all around me. Everything goes black.

"Amy…Amy, can you hear me?" I awake to green gowns and face masks. "Amy can you feel this?" My body cringes as ice-cold pain shoots through every vein in my existence. Everything goes black.

I awake to a terrifying realization: There is no pain in my legs. There is no pain from my waist down.

Amy, you were in a car accident. Your mother tells me you were on your way to the mall to meet your friends. "Do you remember?" A jumbled assortment of my family, doctor, therapist, surgeon, guidance counselor, grief counselor, and family therapist try to encourage me. "Amy, remember it will take time. This doesn't mean you can't live a fulfilling life."

My therapist explains my T8 contusion as if reading from a script. Several spinal nerves responsible for sending impulses to my brain are no longer connected. I lack lower motor control. I am unable to walk. I require a catheter at all times because I lack bladder control. I will have physical therapy to avoid atrophy of my leg muscles. I will need a wheel chair to get around. I learn that improper use of the wheel chair can result in a dislocated rotator cuff. The numbness of my therapist's voice evokes tears from my eyes. Everything goes black.

Three months crawl across my consciousness. Every morning begins with a feeling of regret. Every morning begins with a memory of my carelessness. My mind plays the lyrics that are forever carved into the recesses of my existence:

"Don't worry about the future; or worry, but know that worrying is as effective as trying to solve an algebra equation by chewing bubblegum. The real troubles in your life are apt to be things that never crossed your worried mind. Don't stress about the small things, the things you should worry about will just hit you." ☼

*Baz Luhrmann, Sunscreen. Mary Schmich, a staff writer for the Chicago Triubune, first wrote these words in June 1997. Her article was titled, "Advice, like youth, probably just wasted on the young." Later that year the words appeared as an internet hoax claiming to be the commencement address given at MIT in 1997. The words caught the attention of Austrian film director Baz Luhrmann who purchased rights to the words in 1999 and turned them into a song. "Sunscreen" was the most requested song played on morning shows that year.

Michelle LeBlanc is a Bio Med graduate student working on her Master's degree at Barry University, Miami Shores, Florida.

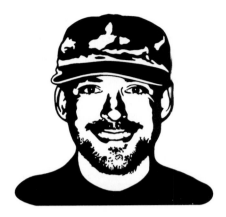

The Happiness Paradox

By Mort Laitner

Seven years after the Great Collapse, they popped up--like McDonald's in the fifties, Blockbusters in the eighties, Jenny Craigs in the nineties and Starbucks in the first decade of the new millennium. They sprouted in city shopping centers, with Crayola-colored store front windows, plastered with sunflowers and sunshine. Happy faces bounced across their window panes. Four words painted in psychedelic oils with 18 inch lettering transfixed my eyes, "ENTER AND GAIN HAPPINESS." Those words were reminiscent of the late sixties where they were found on head shop windows or on Hari Krishna's doors.

I could not resist the aura emanating from the window art. It sucked me in and I needed help.

The last time I had been truly happy eludes me. I felt depressed for days after having left my rose-colored glasses in Applebee's. I remembered reading on their menu, "Happiness begins with dessert." So I tried it. The Applebee's dessert left me empty—just as if my meds were either wearing off or not working at all.

I cat-crawled to the center's portal in need of a natural high.

The sign at the entrance door read:

Learn how to stay happy on a tight budget.
We promise to help you enjoy life with fewer toys.

We'll teach you how to manage your free time as well as your life.
Find inner tranquility with the help of our professionally-trained staff.
We are committed to making you happy.
Your happiness will rub off on your loved ones.

I heard similar words on the Oprah Show. Her guests calmly voiced their messages on enjoying life with less material wealth. Now corporate America was going to make a buck off of this scheme. I wanted to get mas por menos, more of life's happy experiences while paying less pocket money.

I pulled the door open, as Claude Debussy's Claire De Lune filled the room. Each note penetrated my ears and drove into my soul. The sweet aroma of burning incense crept up my nostrils. The clinic staff was draped in white lab coats. Some of the coats were fashioned with red, yellow and blue polka dots as if they were taken off a loaf of Wonder Bread. Each employee wore a smile and blue name tag with their first name and job title printed on it.

I read the greeter's name and title, Jenny—Happiness Counselor. This pretty, twentyish blond with black plastic glasses said, "Good morning sir, how can we help you?"

"I'd like to become a member of your happiness tribe," I replied.

She half-heartily giggled at my feeble attempt at humor. Jenny handed me an iPad 8, "Please answer 'all' the quality-of-life and the medical care questions and return the pad to me so I may assign you your own happiness specialist. He will explain to you our program and your happiness index score."

I pondered, was Jenny really happy? Then I went to work for the next thirty minutes answering all one hundred questions. While typing in my answers, I studied the two patrons seated across from me.

One was a six-foot tall, skinny, twenty-something, unshaven male with nicotine stained fingers and unruly lock of jet-black hair. He wore a tattered green and orange football T-shirt with the name of some defunct college program emblazoned on it. His sunken eyes and his state of wear depressed me.

Seated next to Slim sat a fortyish year-old female. On her arm she wore a cat tattoo and a T-shirt in which three cats played with a ball of yarn. She was a bit overweight, a bit homely and looked as unloved as a gila monster.

They sat in silence. My heart wondered whether these two ever find happiness.

The queries on the iPad reminded me of the books I had read on the indexing of countries by how happy their populations were. I wondered if my score would fall off the chart. How many sessions would it take before my score would weigh-in as happy.

Handing the pad back to Jenny I asked, "What is the lowest score you have ever seen?"

"It's not today's score that matters. It's the score you reach in the next few months that counts. Please take one of these twenty week program guides and read it. It will help you make your decision about joining us."

I reached out to accept the brochure and accidently touched Jenny's hand.

Acting like the touch never happened I replied, "Thanks Jenny, I'll review them as I wait for my counselor."

Sitting in the waiting room, I scanned the testimonials on the wall. These large photos of young and old, male and female with their perfect smiles and perfect teeth all praised the program:

"It was the best money I ever spent, I have never been happier."

"I couldn't believe my luck in finding Happiness. My life couldn't be better."

"This program really works! You have got to give it a chance."

"Why be depressed? Find happiness in our loving hands."

These testimonials reminded me of my need to hit the mens room.

"Jenny, can I have the keys to the bathroom?"

"Sure," she responded as she handed me the keys. This time our hands did not make contact.

I walked and read the center's three clear plastic aluminum-framed posters lining the wall to the restroom:

"What is the meaning of life? To be happy and useful. —Tenzin Gyatso, the 14th Dalia Lama"

"There is only one happiness in life, to love and to be loved. -George Sand."

"No one is in control of your happiness but you; therefore, you have the power to change anything about yourself or your life that you want to change.- Barbara deAngelis."

I contemplated each message. I recalled what I learned in college—happiness is a strange phenomena. It does not obey normal principles, which means that happiness can not be acquired directly. It can only be acquired indirectly. My professor called it something like the "paradox of hedonism."[1]

Returning to the waiting room, I felt conflicted. I placed my reading glasses on and started to review the Happiness twenty-week brochure.

I read:

Week one

Understanding your state of mind, role playing and keeping your diary.

Week two

What is happiness? Why are you sad? Your objective is to change your behavior.

Week three

Define your personal pursuit of happiness. YouTube and musical auditory exercises.

Week four

Choose happiness! Only you can make it happen. Make it your goal.

Week five

Happy foods make happy people. Your diet counts.

Week six

How to give and receive massages, the power of the human touch.

Week seven

Awaking all your senses. Sensory exercises.

Week eight

Time to smell the roses. Diary review.

I stopped reading as the door separating the counselors from the clients swung opened. Counselor Greg greeted me with a Texas-sized smile, handshake and bear hug.

"Come on in buddy, I'm going to teach you a new path to happiness."

---

[1] *Sidgwick, Henry. The methods of ethics. Indianapolis: Hackett Pub. Co., 1981.*

Still trying to catch my breath, I followed Greg to his office.

"Buddy, have a seat and make yourself comfortable. I want you to know our center is a leader in happiness research. You're in the epicenter of the field of positive psychology. At the Happiness Center we apply the scientific method to your issues. Our scientific field is growing by leaps and bounds. Happiness is no longer a fuzzy concept that your parents talked about. With our computer models we can craft you an individualized happiness program, with personalized apps for your everyday use. This center will study your well-being. We monitor your positive and negative emotions. I have reviewed your happiness index and we have a serious amount of work ahead of us. We have had people with lower scores than yours and they have found a better, happier life. Based on your score, I'm going to recommend you sign up for the twenty week program. Every week we will meet at least twice and go over your progress. I'll give you new exercises and techniques to follow and after every session we will tabulate your happiness index. While you were in the waiting room did you get a chance to read the brochure concerning our twenty week activities program handout?"

"I read some of them. It is a pretty interesting list of goals and objectives. What's your success ratio?" I asked.

"Most of our clients move from their state of mild depression to the level of moderate contentment and a good twenty percent make it the full-blown intense joy."

"Wow. That's pretty amazing. How much is the twenty week we program?"

Greg looked me straight in the eyes and without a blink said, "Six hundred dollars. It's a lot of money in our present day economy, but who can put a price on a happy life? In addition you receive:

One Choose Happiness T-shirt;

One hundred happy face stickers which you place around your environment to constantly remind you of the good things in your life;

Plus, a ten week supply of Happiness bars, our scientifically-formulated nutrition bar that will alter your mood within minutes."

Greg smiled and continued, "You look convinced, ready to make the change and invest in your future."

I smiled and started to reach for my wallet. Pulling my wallet out of my pants, it flipped opened and I saw the picture of my cat. Greg's spiel collapsed. The picture of my cat popped into my head and I remembered something else I learned in college. "Greg, happiness is like a cat, if you try to coax it or call it, it will avoid you. It will never come. But if you pay no attention to it and go about your business, you'll find it rubbing against your legs and jumping into your lap. It's a paradox. I'm sorry, I'll think about your program, but I'm not joining."[2]

I stood up and walked to the door realizing that money can't buy happiness, but it can buy an education. ☼

---

[2] *Bennett, William J. – A similar quote was written by Henry David Thoreau, "Happiness is like a butterfly: the more you chase it, the more it will elude you, but if you turn your attention to other things, it will come and sit softly on your shoulder."*

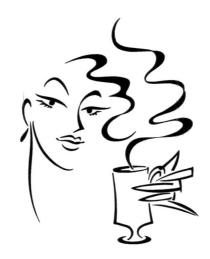

Distractions

By Angela Agazarm

"What can I get for you today?" the barista asked. It was the first time I had visited the new coffee shop in town. I realized immediately that this might, unfortunately, be the happening place in my hometown.

"A mocha caramel latte, whole milk, extra chocolate," I answered. I checked my bag, making sure I had brought everything I needed to study what was the bane of my existence and the key to my acceptance into dental school: neuroanatomy.

"Tall or grande, ma'am?"

"Grande, please."

I found a quiet seat, maneuvering through the teenage crowds and small business meetings. I took out my laptop, headphones, and every highlighter color ever made. I was ready to dive head first into my studying. I did not consider whether the tables next to me had noticed my obsessive compulsive disorder as I re-wiped the table and perfectly stacked each pile of note cards from my backpack. I was fully determined to master Dr. Long's unbearable midterm and overcome my 88.9% average.

I was in the middle of writing out my next note card when I heard someone say, "Studying huh?" That sounded like a pathetic attempt to start a conversation I thought to myself. I looked down and assessed my studying demeanor. I appear focused right? My headphones were visibly in and to the best of my knowledge I didn't look easily approachable.

I tried not to reprimand the older man for rudely interrupting me while I was working. Instead, I replied, "Yes. Would you like to study for me?"

Usually I am good at assessing the irritability probability of surrounding people. However, I hadn't noticed this man when I sat down. I looked at his table and saw a 24-count Crayola box of colored pencils, drawing paper, and the newest version of the iPad. He wore shorts, loafers, and one of those fishing shirts with the netting inside that prevents you from overheating. He seemed retired and bored, but annoyingly chipper.

"I wish I took more pride in my studies when I was a student," he said.

Oh gee here we go. I am not going to get anything done today, I thought to myself. I stayed focused on my laptop, hoping to signal that this was not a good day for small talk.

"What are you studying?" He chimed.

"Me? I am studying neuroanatomy," I said. "Right now I am learning about the ten major cranial nerves."

"That's great. I love how wonderful the body is made. It is fascinating to see how everything works together," he replied.

Well maybe one day I will know, I thought to myself, *but I guess attempting to study here was a bad idea*. I started cursing my bad luck in my head. Why is it that every time I finally get to study, something totally and completely random happens?

"I used to teach and counsel, it was easy to tell the good students from the uninterested ones," he said. "Young lady, where do you live and what do you want to study?"

I reluctantly replied, "Well I am from here actually. I used to go to high school on Ridge Road. Right now I am studying to go to dental school."

I half smiled hoping that would be the end of his desperate need to talk to someone.

"That's wonderful, that is a good school, but I don't hear of too many that go on like you have. Good for you!" he said.

"Well thank you."

Ok, this isn't going to stop, is it? I looked around to see if this was annoying to anyone else and as I did, I noticed a beautiful glass butterfly hanging from the window. I was immediately reminded of my grandmother who always had butterfly trinkets in her house and how she always taught me to respect people and to always show love.

I asked him about his project and what he was working on. In no time we had touched on every topic under the sun, including boats, motorcycles, politics, history, religion and, of course, family.

He had two boys my age that he tried to keep in touch with around their busy lives. I told him that I was one of nine children. We finally exchanged names. He was Harvey Minton from Gainesville. As I talked to him, I realized how nice he was and how much I had learned from just 30 minutes talking with him.

I started to pack up my things, I was going to try and see if the library had died down enough to study there. I decided to put another order in for a coffee before I left. I asked Mr. Harvey to excuse me for one second and I told him that I would be right back.

As I walked back to my seat, I noticed Mr. Minton had left. All of his stuff was gone and he hadn't even said a word. It seemed so odd to me that after all of that he would leave without any sort of goodbye. *Well that seems like my luck, I thought, just as I was packing up, he left.*

I looked down and realized there was a folded-up, hand-written note. On the outside read, "Dear Dedicated Student." As I anxiously peered inside, a business card fell out. I picked it up and read, "Dr. Harvey Minton, Assistant Dean of Admissions, University of Florida College of Dentistry." On the back was written, "It was a pleasure meeting you." Inside the note, Dr. Minton had written, "Thanks for taking the time to talk with me. Never underestimate the impact of kindness. Good luck on your test and God bless you always."

Angela Agazarm is a student at Barry University in Miami Shores earning her Masters in Biomedical Sciences. She graduated from the University of Florida College of Agriculture and Life Sciences and is a member of Golden Key International Honor Society.

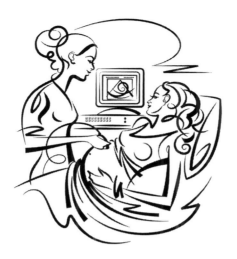

Welcome To Motherhood

By Katie Amrein

In pitch black my clock illuminated the room and in bright green it read 3:00 am, 4:12 am, 5:45 am. I finally awoke an hour before my alarm was set. After a night of restless sleep, I had this mystical energy coursing through my body. The only other time I have this feeling is when I have too much caffeine or a new crush. As I poured myself four 8-ounce glasses of purified water, I pondered on the past four and a half months of my life. A small human being was growing in my had-too-much-for-lunch-looking belly.

Yes, it was a little miracle inside me. That's great and all, but what I'd been losing sleep over since the day I found out I was having a little bundle, was the sex. Forget all the embryology – does it have a penis? Today was the day to put it all to rest. My first ultrasound.

Although the goal of this routinely second trimester ultrasound was labeled "fetal anatomy assessment," it served a different purpose for me. I became obsessed with the sex of the baby – it's all I could think about. I bought fertility crystals and rubbed them on my belly praying to the fertility gods to give me a boy. I constantly visualized my baby boy in baby converses, a mohawk hairdo and surfer tees. Friends and strangers even fueled my imagination by commenting, "Oh you're holding him low, it's definitely a boy."

My esthetician, who has a gift in reading energies, even told me, "It's going to be a boy." I was positive my dream of having a baby boy was certain. I couldn't wait for swim meets, track meets and soccer games.

I let out a big "Ahhh," three out of the four required glasses down. Still feeling charged I woke up my mother, who flew in from North Carolina for the big news release.

As we left for the doctor's office, I was suddenly aware that my high was wearing off. In a sweet motherly voice my mom asked, "How do you feel?"

I spat back with, "Why does everyone keep asking me that! I'm fine I just have thirty-two ounces of water in my bladder and have to pee." It was a silent trip after that.

Once in the office we quickly became two anxious little girls awaiting their turn with the all knowing ultrasound technician. I had read that the less air in your bladder the better the technician can see the baby so I continued to chug sixteen more ounces of water while waiting.

"Katie," a lady in bubblegum pink scrubs called out. We were finally chosen to go where so many other waddling pregnant ladies had gone before. My mother and I jumped up and followed her under the florescent lighting. After a few pleasantries with the tech, I remembered that this was her job and she obviously wouldn't be under the same giddy spell.

Looking up at the generic landscape mural on the ceiling I fell into a comfortable state and braced myself for the first meeting with my baby. The technician applied the warm, gooey gel onto my belly and away we went. I tried to act interested in the numerous measurements ensuring that my baby was the correct size in the correct places but really just wanted to say, "Is there a penis?" I kept quiet and with a more than full bladder I patiently waited.

But what I wasn't expecting was the heart. This beautiful baby had a fully functioning heart, including ventricles and chambers. Watching the screen I saw the valves open and close and it was at that moment a powerful feeling overtook me. Replacing my adrenaline rush from earlier I was in a serene state feeling awakened, strong and in tune with my body.

"Welcome to motherhood," I said to myself. I wiped away a small tear. Out of the corner of my eye I saw my mom doing the same.

The sonographer then asked the magical question, "Would you like to know the sex of your baby?"

With a big smile I replied with a soft yes. She wiggled the wand around my belly for a few seconds before she said, "It's a girl."

I was quiet and let the tears run down my face. I was in a different dimension. She could have told me I was having an alien and I wouldn't have cared. All I could think about was the image of her small heart beating on the screen. The life I created, my baby girl.

Katie Amrein is a student in the Biomedical Sciences Masters program at Barry University in Miami Shores, Florida.

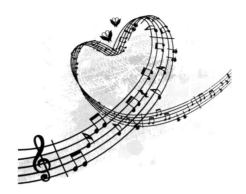

You are Beautiful

By Mort Laitner

As I pulled my luggage through Fort Lauderdale's international airport's vestibule, the automated glass exit doors swung open, chimes rang out and a female voice called out to me. "You are beautiful."

I stopped to listen for more. Not hearing another word, a smile broke across my face as I realized two things:

That the female voice was as automated as the glass doors;

And that I had not heard those words, "You are beautiful" from a female in a long time.

The vestibule's automated doors shut behind me. I entered the sauna known as South Florida. I looked back at the exit and mouthed my appreciation to that anonymous female and the creative artist. "Thanks for the compliment. I needed those words. You are also beautiful."

I walked to my car thinking about the beauty of the airport filled with collages, sculptures, photographs, quilts, paintings and sound art. I had just tasted an audio work-of-art that made my travel experience more pleasant. It changed my mood in an airport, and that is a healthy experience.

I laughed thinking about the first piece of "sound art" I encountered as a child—the self-inflating Whoopee Cushion. This Talking

Vestibule and that Whoopee Cushion were clear voices of the world's best medicine---laughter.

On the drive home, my brain kicked into high gear wondering how prevalent sound art was in the field of health.

After dinner, my computer began buzzing with information. I learned that Jim Green* was the sound artist at the Fort Lauderdale International Airport. His works include laughing escalators, talking fences and talking drinking fountains. His goal is to create socially interactive experiences between his art and the public that surprises and humors.

The rest of my search was almost fruitless. I found an agent pushing sound art for medical centers. I found no hospital, health center or health department using sound art to keep their patients happy and healthy.

I wondered when, if ever, I would be able to compliment a health administrator, who had installed some sound art in their facility elevator, escalator or vestibule with Green's loving words, "You are beautiful." ☀

*JimGreen.org

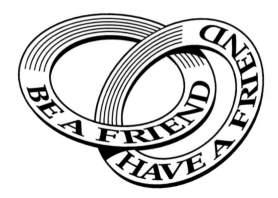

Boom-Shacka-Lacka!

By Deborah C. Pollack

After her divorce Lila could barely get out of bed in the morning. Her husband of fifteen years had asked for a divorce seven months ago to "find himself." However, Lila learned he had been regularly finding himself with his secretary for the past two years. So, Lila found herself sleeping till 11:00 AM, then 12:30 PM and finally till two in the afternoon. She considered swallowing a bottle of sleeping pills but remembered from reading Dorothy Parker's "You Might as Well Live" that drugs caused cramping. Nonetheless, Lila often considered committing suicide.

As she rose from the solace of a deep sleep one afternoon she groggily looked around the brightly-colored *Provence*-style yellow and blue bedroom she once shared with her husband. The room's cheeriness belied Lila's dismal feelings. It would be so much easier if she could slip back into her unmade bed—so inviting, so warm and safe—and stay there forever. But she forced herself to shower, dress, and keep her appointment with a psychologist her older brother insisted on Lila seeing.

For the past seven months Lila had felt a persistent lump in her throat and her skin was constantly dry and cold. When she missed her periods during those first months of agony, she thought she was pregnant. Morosely she drove to a drugstore in the next town and purchased two pregnancy tests. As she walked out of the store, a young Latino man exclaimed, "Why are you so sad, beautiful one?" She didn't answer but weakly smiled at him. At least she wasn't invisible.

She feared she would have a baby that looked like her ex-husband but both pregnancy tests were negative. Five months later, she still wasn't on schedule.

"Come have lunch with me," her close friend, Joanie offered one day.

"No, that's OK," replied Lila.

"Nonsense. You have to get out of the house. Don't worry, I'll cheer you up, I swear," the blond-coiffed, petite Joanie insisted.

Joanie's Mercedes pulled up the graveled driveway and she honked the horn. It was nice to get out, Lila thought as she left the house—something to do instead of weeping alone.

As they rode to a local café, Lila looked somberly at her friend and said "I'm not going to make it."

"Don't be ridiculous! You'll make it," Joanie declared. She then prattled on about a two-year affair she was having with a married man.

Lila wanted to strangle her and scream "Shut up! Don't you see what you are doing to me?" but she merely questioned, "What about his wife?"

"Oh, I really like his wife. He'll never divorce her but that's fine with me."

This created a deeper pain in Lila's heart and the lump in her throat grew larger.

When her brother insisted that Lila get help, she balked.

"I am not going to a shrink!" she vehemently snapped. "And I refuse to take any of those happy pills. They have too many side effects." Ironically, she cared about side effects while simultaneously wanting to end her life.

"Look, you are sleeping till two in the afternoon and you are constantly depressed. You need help to get yourself out of this funk. I'm not telling you to go to a psychiatrist and take medication. I'm just suggesting you see a psychologist. I know someone good who helped out a friend of mine and I think she'll help you as well."

Lila eventually conceded, made an appointment and drove to a neighborhood of modest, older homes about five miles away. She parked her white Ford Focus well away from the therapist's two-story small clapboard house and made certain she wasn't seen before approaching it. This was a huge embarrassment to Lila. She didn't want anyone to know she was one of those women who depended on analysis to keep her sane. After she rang the bell, a smallish, attractive woman wearing a brown sweater and khaki slacks opened the door. She warmly said, "You must be Lila," while removing black framed glasses that matched masses of long, curly, un-behaved hair.

"Yes," Lila answered and burst into heaving sobs.

"Come in, Lila," the psychologist said gently. She led Lila through a small living room. "I'm Dr. Caroline Watterson but you may call me Carol. Let's go into my office at the back of the house."

Lila must have used an entire box of tissues that day, bemoaning the fact that her husband had left her for a twenty-two-year-old woman. "It's such a cliché," she remarked as she wept.

After a time Carol looked at Lila and said, "Look, I could keep listening to you berate yourself and curse your husband while bawling your eyes out but I see I'm running out of Kleenex. So before you go on I have something to share."

Lila sniffed, dabbed her eyes and asked, "What?"

"Ten years ago my husband left me for another woman. I was exactly like you. I wanted to kill myself but I was six months pregnant. So I decided to live until the baby was born. After she was born I had to nurse her so I decided to wait until she was weaned, fully intending to commit suicide when the nursing ceased. I again waited and by the time I had weaned her I felt better. I no longer had the desire to kill myself and had healed by pouring my love into this child. I'm telling you this because while things are bleak for your now, you have to understand that this will change. You will feel better. Depression is so difficult—I know more than anyone—but it can also be somewhat transient. The fact that you came here for help means you are already on the way to a healthier attitude and a healthier life."

Lila was astonished. She thought that all therapists, while merely listening to what you had to say, would just keep nodding and repeating "uh huh." This offering of a personal disclosure was unbelievable. Lila had an ally here, someone who knew exactly how she felt and that revelation somehow made her feel a little better—but not much. "But I have no child and nothing else to live for either." Lila countered.

"You have yourself. And if you don't love yourself, you have to make something to live for—something to look forward to—something special every day that gets you out of your own sadness until you start loving your life again."

"I have nothing to look forward to."

"Lila, talk to your family, your friends. Tell them to give you something to look forward to."

Lila reluctantly took her advice and told her brother who immediately called on his wife, his best friend, and Lila's close friends to help. That night Lila was invited to a delicious dinner cooked by her brother's wife. The next day her friend again took her to lunch but this time did not talk about her affair with a married man. Instead she focused on encouraging Lila.

The following Friday at 10 AM the telephone awakened her.

"Lila" a jovial, husky voice said. "You are coming out with me tonight."

Lila recognized the voice of her brother's best friend—a true "larger than life" lovable character named Rudy who knew Lila from the time she was six.

"But Rudy—"

"No buts—you are coming out with me and I'm introducing you to lots of my single friends. And we are going to dance. Boom-shac-ka-lacka!" (Rudy always said Boom-shacka-lacka to emphasize a highly important statement.)

Lila could not refuse him. She summoned the mental strength and energy to style her hair, pick out a suitable dress and apply makeup. Something she had not done in months. That evening Rudy rang the bell. Exhausted, Lila opened the front door and there he was—six foot two, with a slight paunch, lively brown eyes, olive dimpled cheeks, and a smile as bright as a shaft of light from heaven.

"You look knocked out!" he exclaimed.

Well, I guess that's better than knocked up, Lila thought. "Thanks Rudy." she responded wistfully.

He helped her into his red Mustang and they drove to his club, an elegant members-only establishment in the center of town. They drank, ate, and Lila met Rudy's friends—all up-scale profession-als—who were noticeably attentive to her.

Around nine-thirty as throbbing music began to play, Rudy an-nounced "Now we dance! Boom-shacka-lacka!"

Lila hadn't danced in fifteen years.

"I've forgotten how."

"Bull! Just walk to the beat—like this." Rudy expertly showed her and she followed.

This routine of family and friendly support went on for three weeks along with visits to Lila's psychologist. Shortly thereafter, one morning Lila awoke eager to be on time for her appointment with Carol. Lila needed much less Kleenex that day and looked forward to getting back to work at her previous job as a marketing director and building a better life. She thought it was miraculous her em-ployer still wanted her after seven months of her absence. She also had a date the following Saturday with one of Rudy's friends.

Lila would always be grateful for her brother, her friends, and of course, Carol. But, she especially cherished Rudy who lifted her from sorrow by showing her pure joy. Boom-shacka-lacka! ✧

Deborah C. Pollack is an art dealer and author from Palm Beach, Florida, who has written the critically-acclaimed Orville Bulman: An Enchanted Life and Fantastic Legacy *and* Laura Woodward: The Artist Behind the Innovator Who Developed Palm Beach. *Articles include those in forthcoming magazines, such as* Antiques and Art Around Florida, The Challenge *(the magazine of the Brain Injury Association of America), and* Tequesta.

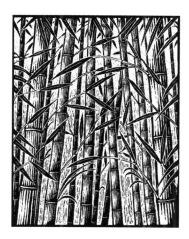

From Where
We Came

By John Dinh

The front door of my house was thrown open at midnight as men charged through to seize my brother. These strangers blindfolded, hand-cuffed, and took him away with no explanation. I did not see him for two weeks. As long as my family still lived under the communist system in Vietnam, more members of my family could be taken away at a moment's notice. Vietnam began to represent captivity as two more of my brothers were imprisoned for five years and my brother-in-law for thirteen years. When I became pregnant with my first child, my husband and I decided we had to leave. No one had a right to break apart my family anymore. My oldest brother, Hai, was already safe in the United States since he was an international student. My husband and I could be safe too if we could get out of Vietnam and get into contact with Hai. Yet, I never imagined how much strength, patience, and faith it would take to leave Vietnam and start a new life elsewhere.

My husband and I had attempted several times to escape to no avail. We eventually learned that a group of thirteen people were planning to escape by boat to Thailand. In the middle of the night, we hid in bushes as we made our way to the neighboring town to reach the boat. Floating on the river for three days, we reached the cape of Cau Mau in the Pacific Ocean, only to be found by police. At six months pregnant, I knew I could not endure any torture and prayed that the police would have mercy on us. Somehow, someone heard me. Instead of arresting us, the police only warned that there was an impending storm and let us go.

After the storm passed, we continued our journey to Thailand. We were only able to use the small seven-horsepower engine during the night when the temperature was cool enough to allow it to run longer. By morning the engine would overheat and shut off. Six days on the ocean passed. We ran out of food, water, and gas. Our boat was ambushed by Thai Pirates. I feared for the worst as I remembered stories of women being raped, captured, and sold by such treacherous people. We were fortunate enough that they only stole our material possessions. We just ran out of money. No land was in sight as we floated aimlessly in the ocean. Now, we ran out of hope. When we sighted another ship, we were so desperate for help that we disregarded the chance that members on that ship could be hostile too. I cried out loud for help. Again, someone heard me.

The captain and crew invited us onto their ship. They fed us for five days and agreed to lead us and our boat near the coast of Thailand. They could not bring us too close to land as there were penalties for harboring fugitives. When we were dropped off, the waves were too big for us to row to shore. We kept trying and trying, but our boat seemed to be going nowhere. I called out to shore in hopes that someone would notice us when suddenly a boy from our boat fell into the water. When he emerged, we realized the water only came up to his shoulders. Someone heard me. Excitedly, we all jumped out of the boat and walked to shore. After fourteen days surrounded by water, I smiled at the site of my feet covered with soft, white sand.

We resided in the refugee camps in Thailand during the next three months in miserable living conditions. After food had grown scarce, my weak body was unable to sustain the growing baby within me. Starvation began to set in. My legs suddenly gave way, and I fell to my knees. My hunger forced me to slowly start picking weeds and grass from off the ground. Unexpectedly, a woman grabbed my arm and took away the weeds from my hand. Cautioning that these were not good for me or the baby, she kindly brought soup and rice for me to eat. However, my body rejected the food as I developed severe diarrhea. The woman's husband found a Swedish associate who worked for the camp to give me an IV. When I recovered, we were transferred to another camp.

Within the camp in Chonburi, my beautiful daughter Vy was born. Yet with another mouth to feed, the food and clothing supplies were running especially low. Vy became deathly ill with a high fever, but I had no medicine to help her. I learned that the refugees were to be transferred to another camp in the Philippines. My husband and I took turns carrying our sick child as we travelled once again to a foreign place. When we arrived in the refugee camp in the Philippines, Vy's small, febrile body stopped moving. She would not drink anything, and her eyes simply remained closed all the time. I questioned how I could journey all this way to have freedom for my family only to cradle this fading child of mine. I could not hold back my tears. Surprisingly, someone heard me.

A man, who knew herbal medicine, offered to help me. He used a remedy of ginger and what appeared to be perfume sticks. In ten minutes, I was still staring at the motionless body of my daughter when suddenly I saw life streaming from her again. She urinated and started crying. I never knew I could be so overjoyed by a simple human action. Over the next few hours, her temperature started lowering, and she was finally tolerating water and milk. The next day, volunteers came to bring us to a clinic, where we finally received adequate medical treatment. We stayed in the Philippines for another five long months until we got a hold of my brother in the United States. He was able to sponsor your dad, your sister, and myself to the U.S.

We understood that this was our opportunity to start a new life for our family. Your dad went to school in the morning and worked at a restaurant at night. I sewed clothes at home to get more income for our family. I must talk about your dad. He is the best father in the world. He is patient, selfless, and unrelenting. I remember he started smoking because he became so stressed. Yet, the cigarettes were not helping anyone. Hai, who had fallen victim to lung cancer, told your dad he had to quit smoking. Your dad realized if anything happened to him, who would help me raise a family that had grown to include three children? Smoking is the only thing that your father ever quit.

After graduating, your dad still could not get a job because of the poor economy. Your dad continued to work at the restaurant with a college degree. I knew we did not struggle to come to the U.S. for us to live day by day as we did in Vietnam. I told your father he must go back to school to obtain a higher degree while I picked up some more odd-end jobs. After some years of living in a cramped house with twelve other people, your dad finished his Master's degree in engineering and was hired by Motorola. We were finally able to afford our own house in Fort Lauderdale, Florida. I could finally see the sunshine through our home—the home where you and your sisters were raised. I know who has been listening and watching over me.

Now, you have heard me. This is from where we came. ✵

John Dinh is a Bio Med student at Barry University who will be attending medical school in the fall.

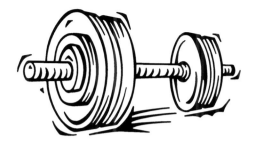

Gluteus Maximus

By Jhelane Vega

I will never forget the day that my boyfriend, George, said to me, "I think I am going to start taking steroids." I was sitting on my cream-colored sectional at a loss for words.

He wanted to shed his body fat quickly, and I knew this was an awful idea. I tried numerous times to talk him out of it. "Honey, not only are anabolic steroids illegal, but there are numerous side effects that come along with prolonged use."

After countless tries to convince George not to take the steroids, it was evident that he made up his mind. That week he started his cycle. George was very content with the results. He worked out daily. He felt stronger than ever before. His endurance skyrocketed, and his confidence significantly increased. Although I was concerned for his health, I was proud of his dedication and newfound motivation to change his lifestyle. Seeing him in high spirits changed the way I felt about steroids. However, I remained concerned.

A week later, I noticed some bruising on George's bottom. This increased my concerns.

Looking at himself in the full-length bathroom mirror, he turned and said, "Babe, this is perfectly normal. It happens to people in the beginning of their cycle. My body will eventually get used to it."

I worried. I continued to keep an eye on the plum-colored spots as they spread. It wasn't long before George came to me and said, "Please take a look at this spot that I have, it feels strange."

I nervously pulled down the backside of his Nike Jordan shorts.

I noticed a raised area that was warm to the touch. I expressed my concern. "George, this is serious! You must see a doctor."

Again, he claimed that it was normal and that his skin might just be tender from the steroid injections. The next few days proved that something was not right. What was once a small rosy spot spread to cover most of George's gluteus maximus. Not only was it warm to the touch, but it was now firm and darker in color.

Friday afternoon, George asked, "Will you accompany me to the urgent care center?"

The waiting area smelled of hand sanitizer and Lysol. After waiting for what seemed like an eternity, George was finally called in and we walked to the back to be triaged and placed in an examining room. Minutes later, the doctor came in to examine George's bottom.

George admitted to beginning an anabolic steroid cycle in hopes to bulk up and eliminate body fat. The doctor advised, "Stop the use of the steroids! Come back in two days for another evaluation."

George was prescribed an antibiotic and told to apply ice to the raised area. He was diagnosed with cellulitis, a skin infection caused by bacteria.

On Sunday, we returned to the urgent care center. Unfortunately, George's condition did not improve. The doctor then prescribed another antibiotic and a medication used to treat an upset stomach. Once again, George was told to return in two days.

Finally, on Tuesday when George visited the urgent care center for the third time, the doctor informed him that his condition had significantly improved but that he was to continue taking his antibiotics until it ran out. It took weeks for all of the evident cellulitis to disappear.

We still do not know exactly how he developed the infection, but we are thankful for having caught it early. If we had waited any longer, George would have had to have the area surgically drained. It is no surprise why anabolic steroids are banned in the United States.

George now lives a steroid free-life. He exercises regularly to maintain his weight, and I have the hardest task in holding my tongue every time I want to say to him, "I told you so!" ☼

Jhelane Vega graduated from Florida Atlantic University with a major in Health Administration. Currently, she lives in Miami and is earning her Master's degree in Health Services Administration at Barry University.

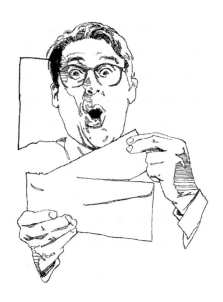

The Envelope

By Phil Reichert

We all waited patiently for the lunchtime festivities. Our office would be celebrating St. Patrick's Day with a pot luck meal. People were dressed in green, and shamrocks graced our walls. But, the celebration never happened. In an unusual twist of fate, everyone was sent home instead. It was like the story of the butterfly that flapped its wings in China and caused a hurricane in the Caribbean. And, it wasn't just our program that was affected. The entire building was evacuated.

It was Friday morning, March 17, 2006, when the Florida Department of Health headquarters in Tallahassee became the unwitting victim of what was either a coldly calculated prank by some evil perpetrator, or the result of some innocent citizen simply attempting to learn if he had come in contact with a communicable disease.

My office was directly across the hall from the mail room. As a program administrator, and due to my proximity, the mail clerk often brought me mail to open that was addressed to the "Department of Health HIV/AIDS Program," but with no specific person or destination available on the envelope. My unofficial job was to open the envelope and help the clerk determine to which individual or program section the letter was addressed.

On this Friday, the clerk brought me a plain white, slightly bulky, standard letter-sized envelope with no return address that was addressed in scribbled pencil to: *Department of Health, Tallahassee, Florida.* There was no zip code and no specific program or person to whom it should be delivered. Since there was no return address, I looked at the postmark. It was mailed in Tallahassee. I found a letter-opener and sliced the flap.

Inside was a not-so-carefully folded Wal-Mart bag with a note attached that stated in the same careless handwriting, *Please test for plague.* I decided not to open the bag, and immediately took the letter and its contents to one of the medical epidemiologists for direction on what to do with this unwanted item. She examined the envelope and looked inside, being careful not to open the plastic bag. We were both very familiar with the aftermath of the anthrax incidents that had occurred soon after nine-eleven. After making a phone call, Dr. Joanne Shulte said, "I wish we had a Ziploc bag to put this in."

I said, "I keep plastic Ziplocs in my office." I retrieved two and we double-bagged it. In minutes, two Capitol Police officers with the Florida Department of Law Enforcement were in our building deciding the next step in this incident. They asked me several questions. *Did you open the plastic bag inside the envelope? What did the note say? Did you notice any white powder?* Since the HazMat team had been notified and were en route, no one would be unsealing the Ziplocs to reexamine the envelope and its contents till they arrived.

The fire alarm sounded. Everyone exited the building, thinking this was simply a fire drill. They left their purses, cell phones, wallets and car keys at their desks in their offices. Fire drills usually lasted about ten or fifteen minutes. Everyone expected to return to their office.

More than three hundred people milled around outside our building as the fire department, the Tallahassee Police Department, the Tallahassee Fire Department, the Leon County Sheriff's Department, Leon County Health Department epidemiologists, the FBI, more FDLE investigators and the HazMat team showed up.

Somehow, smelling the making of a news story, the TV, radio and newspaper people arrived to report on this rare event.

How did I get myself into the middle of this? I was never certain who had the lead as this incident unfolded. Before the police ever arrived, I repeated the sequence of events with my boss, the building guard, my boss' boss and a Leon County Health Department epidemiologist. In the subsequent hours, I told the story at least ten more times. *The clerk brought me the envelope so we could determine where the letter went. I opened it as I would normally do in this situation. I read the note. I took the envelope to Dr. Shulte, our medical epidemiologist. We bagged it. She reported it to the Capitol Police. They evacuated the building. No, I did not notice any white powder.*

After about my fifth or sixth recounting of the events that led to the building evacuation, an FBI agent introduced himself to me and I repeated the same story. He asked if I knew of any employee who might have a grudge against the Department of Health, or some employee or supervisor in our office. I couldn't think of anyone I knew who might be capable or willing to pull a prank like this. It had not occurred to me till that point that someone might have deliberately and truculently attempted to undermine someone in our office, or the Department of Health, in general. I believed from the moment I read the note in the envelope that this event would amount to zilch, nada, zippo.

The incurable optimist that I am, I saw the note in this envelope at face value. I automatically assumed the best case scenario. What if some poor man or woman heard that they may have come in contact with someone who was infected with bubonic plague? He or she might simply place some body fluid (perhaps saliva) into the only plastic bag they had available (a Wal Mart bag) and mail it to the only place they thought could test it (the Department of Health). What did not occur to me until later that day was, if there was some sort of specimen to test in that Wal Mart bag, how would we notify the individual if it tested positive for some communicable disease? Perhaps that was why the FBI agent had asked about the possibility of foul play on the part of the sender.

I watched the HazMat people in their spacesuits carefully handling the envelope I had opened with my bare hands. They used metal tongs as they placed it gingerly into a metal container. The container was put into the rear compartment of an emergency vehicle. I later learned the emergency vehicle sped to the state laboratory in Jacksonville, more than 160 miles, in record time.

Lunch time rolled around. People were still waiting outside the building for someone to make a decision as to whether we would be allowed back inside. We obviously would not be eating the pot luck lunch portions we had brought to celebrate "the day of the Shamrock." The supervisors were told to send their employees to lunch, but they were to return afterward to find out the building reentry status. More than half the people had left their car keys and money in their office. Most people were looking to borrow money, phones and rides from the few who walked outside prepared.

Ultimately, the mail clerk, Dr. Shulte and I were instructed to go home, remove our clothing either outside in our garages, or in a room away from others in our household, place those clothes into a plastic garbage bag and tie it off. Next, we were to shower thoroughly with antibacterial soap. Someone would call us with further instructions.

Two FBI agents came to my house to question me further (Now, *there's* a statement you don't ever want to have to say). I repeated the story for the thousandth time. They were genuinely looking for the name of a person who might have been capable of causing this calamity. It didn't seem as though I was being accused. I think their investigation revolved around speculation that the culprit knew someone in our office would open the letter, and that it would cause alarm.

After my "decontaminating" shower, I received a call from my boss. Our building was closed for the remainder of the day, and everyone was sent home on administrative leave. We got an early start on our weekend.

What lessons were learned from this experience? Always have plastic storage bags on hand, preferably the ones that zip closed. If the fire alarm sounds, walk outside with your wallet, purse, keys, money and cell phone. And, whatever you do, don't open any bulky envelopes with sloppy, incomplete addresses written in pencil that do not have a return address.

In the subsequent weeks, there were people I barely knew from as far away as Miami telling me they had heard about the "letter-opening incident." Odd news travels fast. And, what were the results of the Wal Mart bag that was whisked to the state laboratory to be examined and tested? It turns out, there was no plague or any other communicable bacteria or virus. There was, however, semen and saliva. I had opened the envelope that March 17th, but I am eternally grateful I had left the Wal Mart bag alone. ☀

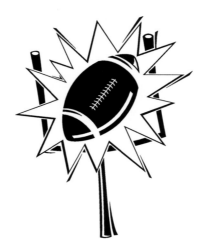

Slip Sliding Away

By Mort Laitner

Climbing back on my Pro Form treadmill, I pause to think, you are a failure, a dismal failure…you bought it…why don't you use it…it has been months since you lost a pound…you're hardly ever using this expensive piece of exercise equipment.

Have you forgotten the meaning of discipline? Have you forgotten your change of lifestyle? You're drinking less water and eating more carbohydrates, no wonder you have regained, how much…five pounds!

Your promises, your commitments and your goals just keep slip sliding away.

Your metabolism comes to a halt. You are no longer burning fat. You are no longer feeling that euphoria of fat melting off your body. You have become a basal metabolist, burning the minimal amount of energy to breathe and to take care of your other vegetative functions. Your lack of exercise and water has decreased your metabolic rate.

As I grasp the treadmill's handrails, my brain yells, wait a minute, maybe it is not all your fault, maybe your lack of success was caused by your body's production of Leptin, the chemical that controls metabolism.

Damn you, Leptin! You're the culprit. You are as evil as my inner child that hides beneath my belly; that cake-eating brat that continues to try to conquer my weak, undisciplined self. Why hasn't my expensive weight loss program warned me about this internal enemy? I guess that divulging that fact may not be in their best interest. How does a weight loss program combat a chemical housed deep within your body?

Well you hardly ever go to that program to get weighed-in. You are a quitter. Your friends warned you, "Your quick weight loss will turn into slow weight gain. You will be like all their other customers with their initial success and their slow return to fat land."

So now the program wants me to "stabilize" my weight after it took me a month just to lose that last pound. "Stabilization," there is a fancy word for "Sucker you're not going to be able to lose another pound."

The program says, "We want you to stay slim, but let's experiment." Now they allow me to eat cake on those "special occasions." That's like giving a heroin addict a taste to remind him of what he is missing. Stabilization means I'm allowed three starches in their daily menu plan. Now the diet counselors tell me, "Cake and starches are okay." Funny, it's not them suffering with each additional pound recorded on the electronic scale.

Damn you weight loss program! What do you have against consistency?

I stop beating myself and the weight loss program up long enough to place the red plastic key on the machine's start spot. I set the speed at 2.2 miles per hour – with no incline, as my legs mechanically move forward.

I grab the remote and click on the TV. My luck, a "look-at-me-see-how-many pounds-I-have-lost" commercial burns into my eyes. I watch as former Miami Dolphin quarterback, Dan Marino, brags about losing twenty-two pounds on NutriSystem. Yeah, NutriSystem the "advanced" weight loss program based on the Glycemic Index. Yeah, everyone watching this advertisement knows what the Glycemic Index is. My highest weight loss number was twenty-one pounds. I wonder what Dan's weight is today. I wonder why he doesn't mention Leptin. I mentally kick myself for my lack of performance. I should have at least tied Marino.

Damn you, Dan Marino, I'm going to beat you. I'm going for twenty-three pounds.

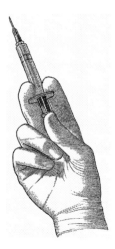

The Fast Life

By Hugo A. Ramirez

I can still remember the first time I saw a hypodermic needle. It made my stomach quiver. The year was 1987 and our family doctor, Dr. Orozco, gave me a shot of penicillin to relive my chronic case of tonsillitis. I remember him saying to my mother, "This problem with his tonsils has been happening too often. The next step will be to remove them." Although the shot of penicillin did its job efficiently, less than a year later my tonsils were removed.

There are two reasons I recall that needle. One, I gave the doctor a hard time when I was asked to drop my shorts and expose my glutes. And two, because after seeing the size of the syringe all I could think of was, "Real Men Don't Cry," a quote from a No Fear shirt I often wore and which made me feel tough.

I am fortunate enough to say that while growing up in Miami I have acquired a good group of friends. The six of us met in the fifth grade gifted program, not long after my first encounter with the hypodermic needle. We remained friends through high school. We all came from good families. What differentiated our group from the rest is that we loved to cause havoc, but we equally took pride in excelling scholastically.

In my sophomore year, worries about Advance Placement Tests

and grade point averages caused my friend Jeff and I to face reality. We both came from single parent homes and we needed to step up to the plate to help our families financially. I took a part time job at a local pizza and sub shop. Jeff got a job at the first place that hired him, a McDonald's.

Jeff was the smallest and scrawniest from our group. At that time he was five-feet five-inches and weighed 130 pounds soaking wet. Although exercise was always a routine with our group, Jeff never seemed to bulk up like the rest of us. Most of the time when the group was involved in an altercation, it was to defend Jeff.

Once Jeff started working at McDonald's things heated up. Jeff would work on weekends and other students from our school would pick on him by being difficult in the drive-thru lane, spitting spit balls at him, and trying to short change him. The constant abuse got to Jeff.

One day at Jeff's house, he called me into his room. As I stood up from the couch in the living room and began making my way, I questioned myself, "What? Another idiot picked on Jeff?" I walked into Jeff's room and he closed the door, only this time he had done something odd, he locked it.

My friend placed his arms on top of his armoire and without facing me said, "I am done with people picking on me and being a PUNK! Brother, I asked you to come here to tell you what I am going to do about this. I spoke to my cousin and he said the best way to get respect is to become HUGE."

"Jeff, we are doing what we should, taking whey protein, weight gainer and working out hard. You will see, soon you will catch up."

I wasn't even able to finish my last word before he yelled at the top of his lungs, "NO!" Jeff turned around with a face full of tears looked at me and said, "Bro, I am tired of this S&@T! My cousin gave me this." In his hands I saw something I had not seen in years, a hypodermic needle. The syringe shook in his hands along with some small glass tubes. Once I saw both objects together I knew what it was.

I told Jeff, "Are you crazy? You don't need to juice to fix your problems. That stuff is dangerous and can hurt you plenty." Jeff and I spoke for a few hours that day. Most of the time, I was trying to convince him not to take the steroid path. Our conversation ended when he told me he had just taken his first shot some hours earlier.

Jeff's decision worried me and because of it, I kept close to him. Jeff started a cycle of 250 milligrams of Testosterone and 100 milligrams of Methenolone Enanthate (Primo) once a week. He assured me that as long as he kept these small dosages for no longer than eight weeks he should not develop harmful side-effects like elevated cholesterol or triglycerides.

As time passed, Jeff transformed into a bigger more muscular person. He quit his job at McDonald's and started a job in the gym where he worked out. Jeff made new friends at the gym. Some of these, so called "friends" counseled him on other steroids to take. Before long, Jeff transformed into an animal and yes, no one messed with Jeff anymore.

My friend spiraled out of control. He started making real money training people in the gym and supplying fools with juice. Jeff went from doing eight-week cycles to sometimes taking steroids all year long. He practically lived with a syringe constantly inserted in his buttocks. Jeff experimented with just about every steroid available. He took Nandrolone Decanoate (Deca), Stanozolol (Winstrol), Trenbolone (Tren), Finaplex(Fina) and an array of testosterones in doses as high as 750 milligrams a week. Jeff worried us all. He drifted from the group and let his grades drop. All he thought of was lifting weights, training clients and making money. Jeff was always a charismatic guy. He soon became a very popular person in all social groups. People from other schools knew him and older people respected him.

Two months before our senior year ended, Jeff struck me with the biggest blow. He decided not to graduate high school and instead get his GED. He had already missed about a quarter of the school year. He said he could use the next couple of months to train, work hard and get ready for the summer. Soon after the news, Jeff began to work for a club promotion group. This group hosted some of the best parties at South Beach's most exclusive nightclubs. Jeff felt he was in the highest point of his life—feeling important when covering the door at the club and choosing who to let in and who not to. Along with this new life came many temptations. In June 1998, my four other friends and I graduated high school. Jeff graduated into a life of fast women, lots of money, alcohol and drugs.

The summer of '98 tore our group apart. Four of my friends moved to Gainesville to attend college and I stayed in Miami. Over the years we kept close contact and they always asked me to fill them in on the latest news about Jeff. I would see Jeff occasionally whenever he was hosting a new party at a club on the beach. Every time I saw him there was something new about him: the Rolex watch, the $500 Hermes belt or the Gucci shoes. I noticed another thing, Jeff kept getting bigger than ever. I came to find out he started taking human growth hormone. At this point I recognized this whole lifestyle had taken the best of him. Although Jeff looked like an ultra healthy person, inside he was ruining himself. Jeff started using hard drugs like cocaine and ecstasy. He told me unbelievable stories about going to weight lifting competitions in Vegas and after the competition staying up for days on end, then returning to Miami and starting the binge where he left off.

I always asked Jeff about his health and if he was getting check-ups. "Your rough lifestyle can kill an elephant," I told him. He assured me he had checked his liver, kidneys, pancreas, blood pressure and also done an STD test. After the last check-up, the doctor gave him medication to regulate his blood pressure.

A few years later I received a phone call from Jeff's mom. She informed me Jeff was hospitalized because he had a seizure. The whole drive to the hospital had me worried with questions. What could have caused the seizure? When I got to the room, I found Jeff with a bunch of tubes coming in and out of him. He looked terrible. He was jaundiced, and I knew right away his situation was grim. The heavy drug and alcohol use, along with his addiction to steroids, had taken a toll on Jeff's liver and kidneys. There he was, my close childhood friend, unresponsive and in a coma. I cried.

It wasn't long after that Jeff passed away due to systemic organ failure. He died at the tender age of thirty. The hardships he experienced as a kid and his inability to cope lead to his downfall. Jeff found the fast and easy way to become muscular, make money and gain respect. If he had taken the harder path, Jeff would have accomplished all these goals, maybe not as fast, but he would still be alive. ✤

Hugo A. Ramirez was born in San Jose, Costa Rica. He attended Miami-Dade College and graduated from Florida International University with a Bachelor's Degree in Health Service Administration. He is currently attending Barry University where he is enrolled in the M.B.A. program with a specialization in Health Service Administration.

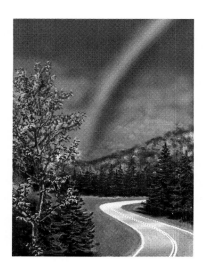

The Colors of My Rainbow

By Christina Martinez

"License and registration please," the officer said. Such emblematic words reminded me of an atypical day seventeen years ago. Here we were again, third time this semester, another usual morning where one of those men my parents told me were "good guys" would stop my mother to give her some blue papers.

"Officer, I apologize. I didn't see the light turn red." For some reason my mother would be mad and crumble the papers. Why did the "good guys" always make her so angry?

It was Friday, so I got to wear my awesome purple PE shirt. We arrived at school twenty minutes past eight, tardy enough to need a late-pass to get into class. Once at the door Mrs. Hernandez, my kindergarten teacher, greeted us while my mother explained our mishap. "That's okay, I'll just need the green copy of the excuse." My mother handed her the copy, to which the teacher once again clarified, "I need the green copy. You handed me the yellow one." I kissed my mom goodbye, as the teacher once more said, "Oh, and for next

Friday, please bring Diana wearing the correct red PE shirt." My mother responded with a smile.

I enjoyed being at school, but the playground was by far the best part. I loved being outside with the pretty pink sky. "When will we go outside?" I asked Mrs. Hernandez.

"It seems like a sunny, beautiful day, but since you are not wearing your correct PE uniform you will not be allowed outside today."

I didn't understand. My shirt looked the same as everybody else's. Instead of being allowed to play in the playground, I was given a coloring assignment and forced to stay inside. Mrs. Hernandez decided to give me a drawing sheet that she had left over from a previous assignment. She gave me the picture with the traffic lights. That was easy. I would paint it fast and still be able to play in the blue doll house that I liked so much. I started coloring immediately, but it took me a while to find the exact colors I needed since all the crayons seemed to be the same color. When I finally finished, I wrote my name and handed it in.

"Can I go play in the blue doll house?" I asked Mrs. Hernandez.

"Yes Diana, you can certainly go play in the PINK doll house." As I was about to run towards the toy corner, she called, "Diana, come here again. Do you remember when you colored this sheet the first time? Are those the colors we said were correct?"

Why was she asking me this? And so many other questions, she kept confusing me.

"Are these the colors you see on traffic lights while you are in the car?"

"Yes. My dad had taught me to be aware of the traffic lights. The one at the top meant ROJO PARA. The middle one was AMARILLO SUAVE. And my favorite, the one at the bottom, VERDE VAMOS."

The teacher kept scolding me. She said, "You need to see a doctor for your eyes."

I couldn't understand. Why was she so mad? I started crying. I didn't want to see a doctor. My eyes worked just fine.

When the school day ended, Mommy came to pick me up, but Mrs. Hernandez decided she needed to talk to her. She explained that a child my age should know their colors. She was concerned about how I could be very good in hard subjects, but still not know the correct colors of the traffic lights. Mrs. Hernandez stated that I had painted blue, grey and purple. She again suggested I be taken to an eye doctor. To all this, my mom replied that those were the exact colors she saw on traffic lights.

Mrs. Hernandez looked confused. My mother gave her a weird smile and explained how she was partially colorblind. She explained all this stuff I didn't understand about how it meant that she lacked the short-wavelength cones, and it made her unable to distinguish colors. She had been warned that she could pass it on to her children, so she had already made sure my vision was working fine.

I was only four years old, listening to something I couldn't understand, but would rationally explain so many things in my life to come. At four years of age this could only make me feel worried that Mrs. Hernandez would never be able to see how beautiful the sky looks in pink. ✲

Christina Martinez is a biomed graduate student at Barry University.

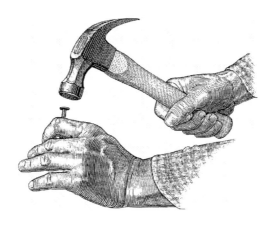

You Nailed It

By Mort Laitner

Lathering my face, I glanced in the mirror and observed my first grey eyebrow hair. It sprouted out of a black forest like a seagull gliding through a flock of crows. I wondered if I should pluck it. This sign of aging made me reflect on the three items resting on the sink—the roll-on deodorant, cologne from Kenneth Cole's Black collection and Old Spice shaving cream. All three products seemed to have lasted for well over two months. They showed no sign of graying. I wondered which would be the first to go.

I remembered smelling Old Spice for the first time in 1960 in Rashkin's Pharmacy. I bought a dollar bottle of Old Spice aftershave for my Dad. I pulled the plastic grey stopper and inhaled the unmistakable sweet odor of Old Spice. It came in a buoy-shaped white glass bottle with a drawing of a clipper ship. On the bottle a strong wind filled the ship's large sails. I recalled the TV commercial where a handsome sailor wearing a blue jacket and a cap swaggers off the ship with a duffle bag flung over the shoulder. His destination is an attractive woman. As I picture the sailor meandering through the streets, I started whistling the catchy nautical Old Spice jingle and remembered the first birthday present I ever gave my Dad.

For a month, I saved my meager twenty-five cent weekly allowance. My Dad seemed pleased when I handed the Old Spice. I said, "Happy Birthday Dad." He replied with a firm hug, a kiss on my cheek and a twinkle in his eye and said, "I love your gift." I nailed it.

That Old Spice year my Dad decided to send me to Camp Alamac. I questioned his selection, but he knew the camp was within walking distance of our home and it served the campers the same hot lunch the hotel guests received. The summer was my father's work-like-a-madman season. Our community grew from a few thousand to over twenty thousand. As one of the town doctors, he rose at six, was in the hospital by eight, back in his medical office seeing patients by eleven and then he did intermittent house calls until it became dark at nine. Camp would keep me out of his hair except for a quick dinner.

So every morning at 7:30 I sucked in the crisp mountain air and walked ten city blocks to camp. I strolled across the railroad tracks whistling, "Someone's in the Kitchen with Dinah" while observing the beauty of small town America. My mind wandered as I daydreamed about fishing while listening to robins chirp and watching them wrestle worms from the ground.

Down Broadway toward the Glen Wild Road, I skipped with my only stops consisting of meeting and greeting fellow campers until I reached the camp.

Life was simple with no worries about satisfying the opposite sex. My goals were limited to pleasing my parents, friends and counselors. I never thought about school.

My daily camp activities were well organized: dodge ball, baseball, soccer, shuffle board, football and punch ball. There were color wars and arts and crafts. With pride I remembered braiding my own key chain lanyard. On rainy days, we played knock hockey or ping pong. Life was fun. Camp Alamac had nailed it.

The Alamac was a fancy Catskills hotel with a small day camp. From June first till the day after Labor Day the hotel and day camp were packed with New York City tourists---city folk and Woodridge, New York campers---country folk. The hotel consisted of a large three story guest house, an Olympic-size pool which was landscaped by fifty-foot maples and our camp building.

A smattering of white Adirondack chairs rested on the green

manicured lawn. The smell of the freshly cut grass filled your nostrils as quickly as an opened bottle of Old Spice. The property gave the appearance of wealth and class--a look desired by those tourists from New York City. They also loved the food. The three C's meant nothing to them. Cholesterol, carbohydrates and calories were "future speak" and the average life span of those tourists was 65 years. A typical Alamac Hotel menu read:

Please make one choice from each course

First course

Chopped liver appetizer with a freshly baked challah or bialy
Gefilte fish with purple horse radish

Second course

Chicken soup with yellow circles of molten chicken fat
floating across its surface
A bowl of borsht with a glob of sour cream partially submerged
in it as if a floating Iceberg in the dark North Atlantic.

Third course

Boiled chicken
Brisket
Both entrees served with carrot tzimmes cooked in honey

Fourth course

Home made:
Apple strudel,
Babka
Rugelach.

No one ever left the table feeling hungry.

When it came to food the Alamac Hotel nailed it.

Forty years after I attended Camp Alamac, my Dad passed away. Under his sink, I rummaged through and examined his toiletries. There stood his shaving cream, his deodorant and to my surprise, my gift, the Old Spice aftershave. I gently picked it up as if it were a valuable antique. I pulled out the stopper and inhaled a whiff.

Memories of my father danced in my head. Based on the weight of the bottle I realized it was full. My Dad had never used the first present I ever gave him. I remembered the twinkle in his eye as I gave him the present and smiled realizing that my Dad had kept my gift for over forty years. ☼

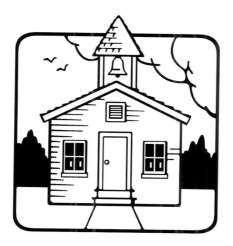

Rash Decisions

By Phil Reichert

en drove from Tallahassee to a neighboring rural county to interview a girl with secondary syphilis.* As he drove to the interview, he wondered what terrible circumstances could have lead to this result. Ben worked in the Sexually Transmitted Disease Control Program for eight years. He thought he had seen it all, but something new always came around that surprised him. This wasn't going to be someone he considered to be one of his normal STD patients, whatever the word "normal" meant. Nope. This was a twelve-year-old girl.

Last week, her mom had taken her to the county health department to find out about that odd rash on the palms of her hands and the soles of her feet. Her daughter's blood test came to Ben's attention that morning. She had not been treated yet because most health care workers don't assume a twelve-year-old is sexually active. So, no one thought her rash was related to an STD.

Ben consulted the department's attorney to make sure it was okay to interview a twelve-year-old with syphilis without notifying a parent. If the client had been thirteen, or older, the law was clear. STD investigators could, and would, talk to clients privately without parents present. If a parent was introduced into the equation, they might prevent the young client from telling the truth about their sexual activity.

Ben's objective was to get the child to tell him names and locating information of all her sexual partners. In the case of secondary syphilis, someone may have infected this girl as long ago as six months. And, according to Ben, there was no telling how many partners she might have infected during the periods of time she was infectious.

Ben arrived at the elementary school where the girl was a sixth-grader. He introduced himself to the principal while showing his identification. "I'm here on urgent public health business. Would you please have this young girl brought to a private office so I can interview her?"

The principal offered, "Why don't you use my office? I have other responsibilities to attend to."

"Thanks," said Ben. "The interview shouldn't take more than twenty or thirty minutes."

As he waited, he imagined the innocent doe-eyed stare of the child as she was called to the principal's office. He anticipated that her fear might create problems finding the person who may have infected her, then getting her syphilis treated. He heard the door open, and his image of the naive schoolgirl was instantly crushed. The twelve-year-old sixth-grader was dressed to impress. She strutted over to the desk in a runway walk that would have made Heidi Klum jealous. Her self-assured stance, her make-up and her skin-tight outfit left little to the imagination, and made her look several years older.

She wondered why she was there. Ben asked if he had her name correct.

She replied, "Yes sir."

Ben thought, sometimes hormones activate early. Looking down at the child's medical record, he discovered the young lady before him was not only infected with syphilis but she had also recently suffered a miscarriage.

Ben introduced himself. "Last week your mom took you to the health department where you had a blood test." The girl nodded in acknowledgement. "That test came back positive showing that you are infected with syphilis. That's a disease that you would have gotten by having sex with an infected person." Ben explained the signs and symptoms.

She whispered, "Yeah, I've had this annoying rash for a couple of weeks now. It's on my hands and my feet. See?" She held up her open palms.

"Those are what we call classic secondary syphilis symptoms," Ben clarified. "And the good thing is we can treat it. Syphilis isn't like AIDS. Currently, there is no cure for AIDS, but this," pointing to her hands, "We can treat and cure." Her body relaxed at this news.

She listened carefully as Ben explained about how she probably became infected and how she could have infected others. Ben asked, "Do you understand what I've told you so far?"

"Yes," she replied.

Ben monitored her eyes to see if her words rang true.

"Do you have any questions?"

"No."

"I need to know the people you've had sex with in the past six months. I reviewed your medical records, and I saw you were pregnant. I need to find the guy who got you pregnant. He needs medicine. I also need to get any others in for testing and for medicine. And, most importantly, you need to have your mom drive you back to the health department today, so you can be treated." The girl identified the boy who got her pregnant and two other sexual partners she had during the preceding six months as students at the county high school. The girl stated, "One of the boys is sixteen, and the other two are seventeen." She described them in great detail and gave Ben their addresses.

After he was finished talking with the young girl, Ben drove to the high school to find the three boys. Now the high school principal gave up his office to Ben for the interviews. After introducing himself he started his normal dialogue, "An urgent matter concerning your health has come to the attention of the health department." He was required to keep things confidential. During the interview with the boy who had gotten this twelve-year-old pregnant, the boy correctly stated the name of his sexual partner, connecting him to her.

This boy said she was sixteen. He either did not know she was twelve and in elementary school, or he was lying. All Ben could do was explain this disease the same way he did with all of his clients. He first discussed abstinence. If that wasn't an option, the person should be in a monogamous relationship. And, if that wasn't an option, then came the how-to-correctly-use-a-condom discussion.

Driving back to his office, Ben thought, Wow. I thought twelve-year-old girls hung out at malls, loved vampires and Justin Bieber. Boy, was I wrong! ☼

* Primary Stage

The primary stage of syphilis is usually marked by the appearance of a single sore (called a chancre), but there may be multiple sores. The time between infection with syphilis and the start of the first symptom can range from 10 to 90 days (average 21 days). The chancre is usually firm, round, small, and painless. It appears at the spot where syphilis entered the body. The chancre lasts 3 to 6 weeks, and it heals without treatment. However, if adequate treatment is not administered, the infection progresses to the secondary stage.

Secondary Stage

Skin rash and mucous membrane lesions characterize the secondary stage. This stage typically starts with the development of a rash on one or more areas of the body. The rash usually does not cause itching. Rashes associated with secondary syphilis can appear as the chancre is healing or several weeks after the chancre has healed. The characteristic rash of secondary syphilis may appear as rough, red, or reddish brown spots both on the palms of the hands and the bottoms of the feet. However, rashes with a different appearance may occur on other parts of the body, sometimes resembling rashes caused by other diseases. Sometimes rashes associated with secondary syphilis are so faint that they are not noticed. In addition to rashes, symptoms of secondary syphilis may include fever, swollen lymph glands, sore throat, patchy hair loss, headaches, weight loss, muscle aches, and fatigue. The signs and symptoms of secondary syphilis will resolve with or without treatment, but without treatment, the infection will progress to the latent and possibly late stages of disease.

Late and Latent Stages

The latent (hidden) stage of syphilis begins when primary and second-ary symptoms disappear. Without treatment, the infected person will continue to have syphilis even though there are no signs or symptoms; infection remains in the body. This latent stage can last for years. The late stages of syphilis can develop in about 15% of people who have not been treated for syphilis, and can appear 10–20 years after infection was first acquired. In the late stages of syphilis, the disease may subsequently damage the internal organs, including the brain, nerves, eyes, heart, blood vessels, liver, bones, and joints. Signs and symptoms of the late stage of syphilis include difficulty coordinating muscle movements, paralysis, numbness, gradual blindness, and de-mentia. This damage may be serious enough to cause death.

(http://www.cdc.gov/std/syphilis/stdfact-syphilis.htm)

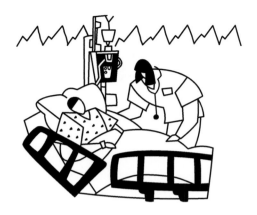

Wasted Energy

By Victoria Guerrero

Working in an ER you become accustomed to hearing horror stories about people coming in and never leaving. My 2:00 PM shift quickly became the kind of shift I dreaded. I spent the entire time running around and never catching up with all my work. By 4:00 PM, Dr. Goldman and I saw seven patients with typical abdominal pain, two patients with nondescript chest pain and one ankle injury.

Then we got a call from the charge nurse saying, "Dr. Goldman, we have a trauma coming in for you. It's a 50 year-old male that lost consciousness while watching the Dolphins game with friends. The EMT noted some facial drooping, slurred speech and motor loss to his right extremities. They are three minutes out."

We ran to the trauma room. Moments later the EMT rolled the stretcher in. The patient vomited violently into the tiny powder blue bags. The nurses were deciphering this man's history from the information that the EMTs gave them and from what they could translate from the patient. They figured out that he had a history of hypertension and was noncompliant with his medication. They also figured out that he had been drinking while watching the game.

During the physical exam, the patient displayed complete motor loss to his right arm and leg. Dr. Goldman decided that he needed to protect the patient's airway and intubate him. He wanted to get a clear head CT scan. His practiced hands slid the endotracheal tube down the sick man's trachea and you could see the slow rise and fall of the patient's chest.

"Get me a chest x-ray to confirm the tube is in the correct position!" Goldman ordered.

We stepped out and continued to see other people whose complaints seemed minor in comparison. A nurse began to search the distressed patient's cell phone to see if he had any family or friends to be contacted.

A few minutes passed when Dr. Goldman received another phone call. "What do you mean the patient is blue?" He slammed the phone and sprinted down the corridor. I ran behind him with my computer on wheels (COW). I was so concentrated on catching up with Dr. Goldman that I didn't see the nurse in my peripheral vision and hit her with the COW.

"I'm so sorry. I think our patient is dying!"

By the time I reached the room, Goldman had removed the endotracheal tube and was attempting to insert a new one. Apparently, while the x-ray tech was positioning the film tray, he moved the patient, pulling the tube out of place.

This time the doctor stayed to watch the chest x-ray. "You're doing it again. I swear to God if I have to reintubate this guy it will be your ass on the line!" he roared. The tech quickly changed his technique and got the x-ray. The endotracheal tube stayed in perfect position.

"Let's get this patient to CT stat please. And get me some blood work with a tox screen! And where the hell is this guy's family?"

The nurse explained that she was unable to find any next of kin and his friends were too intoxicated to drive.

Goldman shrugged his shoulders, "Well, one less crying family to talk to."

We left the patient in his room alone and continued to see our other emergencies while we waited for the CT results.

An hour later the results were up. "Crap, that doesn't sound very good," I said, looking over Dr. Goldman's shoulder to read the CT results. The patient had an extensive brainstem bleed which explained his slurred speech and vomiting. Then we looked at the tox screen. He had large amounts of cocaine in his system.

"Well, I don't feel so bad for him anymore. Let's call the neurosurgeon on call and see what he thinks we should do." Goldman said.

We were directed to speak to the neurosurgeon's Advanced Registered Nurse Practitioner.

"So what's going to happen with that guy in room 50?" Goldman asked the ARNP.

She scoffed, "That guy is a goner! He isn't going to wake up."

"There's nothing you can do?" I questioned. Apparently the bleeding was inoperable which left no options.

The ARNP laughed and said, "He had coke in his system. The guy obviously didn't appreciate his life so why should we waste any more energy on him."

I could not believe what I had just heard. Wasn't she trained to do everything possible to save a life? What if it were her family? Wouldn't she want every doctor, physician's assistant and nurse to stop at nothing to keep him or her alive? Why was this man different?

I never went back to check up on the man in room 50. He was admitted to the hospital and was put under another doctor's care. Whether he died or not, I'll never know. But I do know when I become a doctor that saving lives will never be energy wasted.

Victoria Guerrero has a Bachelor of Science in Biological Science from Florida State University and is currently a graduate student in bio-med at Barry University.

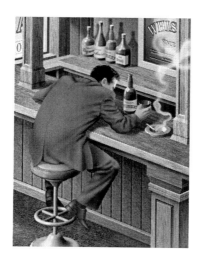

The Cure

By Maya Milman

I t was past midnight on a typical weekday when the phone rang. My younger sister and I had been up watching the Sabrina the Teenage Witch marathon as I picked up the phone:

"Hello?" I answered, wondering who could be calling at this time. "No, this is her daughter speaking."

As I listened to the lady's voice, my face grew white and the hairs on my back of my neck stood up.

"WHAT?" I responded.

***

Sounds intense, doesn't it? Well let's go back to the beginning so that I can properly explain why I am the one answering the phone, why a 16 and 13 year old are up past midnight on a school night, and where are our parents.

You see dear readers, my sister and I are the product of an alcoholic father and an emotionally weak mother. When I was younger, as my father would leave the house to go drinking, my mother would have nothing better to do, but cry her sorrows to me, her 6-year-old daughter. Years have gone by where I had to be the shoulder to cry on for my mother. My father would leave the family for days as he drank himself into different "adventures," as my mother would call it. Many days he came home drunk from a fight with a split lip or bruises all over his face. He was not shy to show us his wounds.

I have a question for you readers, how can alcohol make someone so angry? When my father drank, he turned into the keeper of the peace in his mind, where he decided he should fight for his honor with anyone who has ever wronged him. Every night he would come home and start a war with my mother. In his younger years, my father served in the Russian Army and boxed as a hobby, so you can imagine the type of "discussions" my mother would end up dealing with. My mother was lucky that I, 8 years old by now, was her guardian against my father's drunken outbursts. I grew accustomed to staying up late every night my father was gone, to keep my mother company, calm down my little sister, and be the bodyguard if needed when my dear father finally arrived home. Luckily for all of us, my father would never hit me in his drunken rages, which meant that my mother had the best shield from his blows: my body.

I can go on and on about how terrible my father's outings were, but let me skip to when I was 9 years old and we finally moved to America for the hopes of a better life – whatever that means. My mother was happy to be here because now my father did not have any more drinking buddies, and not knowing English that well, there was a slim chance that he would find new ones. She did not foresee how persistent he or his need for alcohol could be. It turns out that after years of making alcohol the remedy for his stresses, it becomes the only friend he needed. He had no problem going out and enjoying the company of the bottle on his own.

Going out drunk and alone in the neighborhood that we lived in was not just dangerous, it was plain stupid. At least in our country, he was with people he knew who could take care of him. But here, he was alone and on his own. So, imagine the worry my mother felt. Imagine the amount of tears I had to collect staying up and taking care of her. Since my father's obsession had become such a nightly routine, I became a full-time night guard for my mother. Every night my sister and I stood in front of the door crying to our father not to leave just this once. But did that stop him? Not a chance. And it did not matter if it was a school night or the weekend. I was up until my father got home and finally went to bed.

Now readers, you understand why it was a typical school night where we were staying up past midnight. Now we can go back to that phone call.

***

"WHAT?" I screeched as I felt the blood rushing from my head.

"This is Jackson Memorial Hospital calling to let you know that your father has been brought here after a gunshot wound to the face. He is about to undergo surgery." repeated the lady on the other end.

"Oh" I responded, shocked but calm as if I somehow expected this to happen. "Is he going to be okay?"

"We will know after the surgery, but luckily the bullet has missed all major arteries and his chances are good." The woman assured me.

I ran to tell my mother, who was also up waiting for my father. As soon as she heard the news, she sped out to see my father in the hospital, repeatedly screaming:

"He finally found himself some adventure! I knew this would happen!"

***

My father recovered from his surgery. He was able to go home in about a week. The day he came home, I could not look at him. I blamed it all on him.

If only he had listened to me and not left the house, if only he was not stupid enough to try to fight the mugger that had the gun pointed at his head. All the suffering my family endured, all the sleepless nights, and all my mother's tears, I blamed on him. I did not speak to him for months and avoided being in the same room with him.

It took years for me to realize that it was not entirely his fault, and that alcoholism is a disease that took control of his body. I am now 23 years old and am able to forgive my father for everything and be proud of the way he recovered not only from his injuries, but from this ugly disease. He has not drunk like that for four years now and has been trying to rebuild a relationship with his daughters.

It's a typical school night, past midnight and now I spend it working or relaxing, without any worry of an uninvited phone call thanks to my father's cure.

Maya Milman graduated with a BS in biology from the University of Miami and is now a graduate student in the Biomedical Sciences program at Barry University. She hopes to one day attend medical school and become a physician.

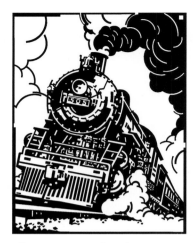

Gambling

By Mort Laitner

Walking in to Dr. Dunn's Office, I noticed his collection of 1940's railroad art. Giant steam locomotives sped through mountain passes. They belched black smoke into the crisp Rocky Mountain air. These powerful monsters gambled with traveler's lives as they climbed steep heights at break neck speeds.

Breaking my trance was the sweet voice of my urologist's receptionist, Terri. She greeted me with her infectious smile, her silky brown hair and her syrupy Southern accent, "Good morning, great seeing you again. How y'all feeling today?"

I remembered how Terri loved to talk. She gave out medical advice like a chain- store pharmacist on a Saturday night.

"All is well," I replied as I twice tapped on my head to ward off evil spirits. "Just here for my annual checkup."

"At your age that's a good idea. Never hurts to know how all your components are operating. Today we got screenings for all parts of your body. We got this PSA test for detecting cancer in your prostate. That's a gland in the lower part of your body." As her eyes scanned to a spot six inches below my belly button, her words chugged along as if she were a train running down the tracks. "The letters stand for prostate-specific antigen. We just draw a little blood from your arm. If your PSA comes back positive then we do a biopsy to see if your cells are cancerous. But before you get screened you got to understand your goals, your fears and your willingness to accept risk."

As I wondered if she had gone to PSA training, I said, "Honey, that's a mouth full of assignments and a lot to think about."

Terri continued, "You don't have to make up your mind today, just sleep on it. You can always come back for the screening."

"Terri, let me tell you a story about a friend of mine who just had his prostate gland removed and he is incontinent and impotent." I queried, "Want to hear how the whole process started? A urology practice gave him free tickets to a pro basketball game in exchange for getting a PSA test."

"But he is still alive—isn't he?" she retorted.

"He is still alive, but he is one unhappy camper. Terri, the man wears DIAPERS! Terri, he lost his MANHOOD!"

Pausing to scratch my mustache I continued, "His urologist's mantra was 'detect early and treat effectively.' His doctor counseled, 'You do not want to be destined to suffer and die.' Before his surgery he read an article calling incontinence and impotence *unpleasant side effects*. His wife calls them disasters. Can you imagine that? He slid down that slippery slope the minute he heard his test results. He could not live with the anxiety of a cancer in his body. He had to remove it. He asked his doctor for surgery to be preformed the next day. You know what he is thinking now? That some cancers are better left undiscovered."

Terri's face reddened as she flung a black clipboard in my direction. The syrup in her voice turned to vinegar as she spat, "Fill out these forms and hand them back to me when you're done."

"Thanks," I replied as I picked up the clipboard which had three sheets of paper pinched between steel and plastic.

Flipping through the pages I scanned their titles:

1. Health Questionnaire Update;
2. Medical Consent Form;
3. Mathematical Probability PSA Screening Consent Form.

This third form intrigued me. Was the government trying to slow the expenditure of limited health care dollars? They knew the risk of death from prostate cancer was only a thousand to one. Was this the urologist's attempt to avoid liability after a patient lost his ability to control his bladder or raise his manhood?

This new form only dealt with PSA screenings. It made me recall handicapping tip sheets at Monticello Raceway. But now instead of wagering on a horse and jockey I would be betting on my life.

I read the form with all the interest of a horse track junkie:

It has been determined that patients should have an opportunity to weigh and respond to health risks by use of mathematical probabilities. Since studies are constantly rendering new statistics we recommend using your computer to update all provided data and by visiting our website to learn more information. Here are the statistics:

90% of men who have a PSA screening have normal results;
10% of men have abnormal results;
Of that 10% there is a 40% chance that a biopsy will show cancer;
There is a 60% chance that the elevation is due to benign causes, such as enlargement.

WE ARE STILL AWAITING RELIABLE RESULTS FROM VALID CLINICAL TRIALS TO PROVE SCREENINGS ARE BENEFICIAL

At the bottom of the form, I rubbed my index finger over the ink:

"I have read this information and after evaluation have decided to: Defer the PSA screening____   Accept the PSA screening____.

I thought about the unstated statistics:
What percentage of men become incontinent?
What percentage of men become impotent?
What percentage of men become both?

For a split second, I stared at the drawings of steam engines on the wall and thought, "I'm not ready to hop on board this locomotive. I knew my goals, my fears and the meaning of black smoke."

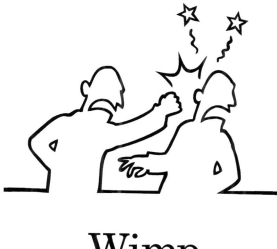

Wimp

By Faraaz Siddiqui

"Wow," I thought to myself.

I was just standing there, arms crossed, leaning against the wall of the venue, staring across the dance floor.

Bodies were everywhere, hundreds of 20-somethings jumping and twisting their bodies left and right to the booming bass and melodic beats coming from the massive speakers on the stage. Surely the club had exceeded capacity, but it was only eleven o'clock.

And yet, with all the commotion around me, I couldn't stop staring at her.

Only a couple hours earlier, I had officially and most certainly blown my chances. We had run into each other. I had been waiting for this moment, this opportunity to finally meet her. A nervous excitement coursed through my body. She was perfect. Her silky-smooth, auburn colored hair framed a smile that could melt even the coldest of hearts. Her caramel colored complexion perfectly complemented the sexy black dress she wore. But what set her apart was the look in her big, hazel-colored eyes, a mixture of loving warmth and compassion with a twinkle of mischief and energy.

I had replayed this moment over in my head hundreds of times. I would casually say "Hello" and then play it cool like Brad Pitt or something, maybe make her laugh a couple times. By that point, she would probably fall in love with me, simple as that.

Of course, things don't ever go as planned.

Instead, my mouth got dry, my hands became sweaty, and my heart raced faster than Seabiscuit.

"Maybe I could pretend to get a phone call and she'd turn around?" I started to reach into my pocket, but it was already too late.

"Hi!" she said, her beautiful eyes perfectly complementing her radiant smile.

"Err…Hi," I awkwardly stammered back. "How…are you?"

"I'm great," she said. "I've seen you around a bunch, but I don't think we've ever officially met."

"Yeah, you're right," I said. And then, my biggest fear came true. I froze. "Uhh…uhh…" I started to look around as she patiently waited for me to say something, anything! I stuck my hands in my pockets, turned my head toward the ground, and then nervously smiled toward her. Awkward silence. It had only been a couple seconds, but it felt like hours. I prayed for something to break the tension. Nothing.

I tried to think of anything I could say, but before I could get the words out of my mouth, I looked up and she quickly said, "Well it was nice meeting you!" still as polite and enthusiastic as ever. Before I could say anything else, she turned around and headed back toward her friends.

I just stood there.

"Fail. Fail. Fail." I thought to myself. "I blew it."

So here I was, lamenting over the catastrophe that had just occurred. If someone stood up and yelled fire in the crowded club, it wouldn't have compared to the chaos that was going on in my mind. Hundreds of thoughts flooded my head: What does she think now? Why did I freeze? Will she ever speak to me again?

I turned away. I had to get my mind off of her. Just as I was walking away, I noticed something out of the corner of my eye.

Amidst the commotion on the dance floor, I looked back toward her and her face was white with fear. A tall, burly man walked toward her, rage in his eyes. I recognized him.

He yelled something at her. Her face wrinkled in confusion. They were arguing. I gazed onward, wondering what was going on.

Suddenly, he cocked back his hand, and with an open palm, his grizzly hands swung forward across her face. Her head swung to the side and she immediately grabbed her left cheek. My jaw dropped. I looked around in amazement. Had anyone seen what I had just seen? The bass of the speakers continued to blare. There was no record screech. There wasn't even the slightest indication that something so shocking had just occurred. Nobody noticed?

I could feel my mouth getting dry, my palms getting sweaty. I started to feel a pain in my stomach. Nobody had seen that?

I had to do something. I summoned all the courage I had in my body and walked toward them. I pushed my way through the bodies of college students dancing with each other. I couldn't just let that happen to her without doing something.

Tears streamed down her face as she looked up at the behemoth looming above her. What a monster. Fear replaced the warmth and enthusiasm I had seen in her eyes only a little while before.

I clenched my hand into a fist and with one swift motion, struck the big man's face. I winced as the pain coursed through my hand. His body slumped to the ground. I knocked him out cold. I turned my attention toward her. She looked at me in amazement. I was her prince charming.

But none of that actually happened.

I rubbed my eyes, and stared on in amazement. I had been daydreaming. I stood there motionless, paralyzed by what I had just seen. I did nothing.

She quickly got to her feet and ran out of the building, only looking back to make sure he wasn't following her. Her assailant's face had changed. He couldn't believe what he had just done. He stared at his hands. They seemed almost foreign to him.

He looked around, embarrassed at what he had just done, and for a moment, our eyes met. He knew I knew. He knew I had seen everything. I could see the fear in his eyes, pleading for me to keep quiet.

And all I could do was stand there. ☀

Faraaz Siddiqui is a student at Barry University in the Biomed program working on his Master's degree.

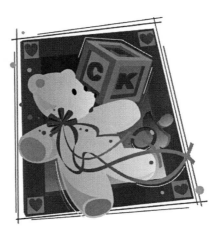

The Test

By Yara Massinga

"Anything yet?" It was the fourth day of hearing my fiancé ask the same question.

"No, not yet." I replied trying not to sound worried. Even though he knew I was. It was times like these that I hated that he knew me so well. I was late. I was never late, early at times, but never late.

"You should probably just go take the test, so you can stop worrying."

"I don't need to take the test! It's probably nothing. I mean... I have just been really stressed lately with apartment hunting, moving, and class. Besides, people are late every day, and it turns out to be nothing." I was trying more to convince myself than him of the obvious cause. "I'll do it tomorrow, I promise. I love you and will talk to you tomorrow."

I hung up the phone, laid in bed, hugging my pink teddy bear. It was the first gift he ever gave me. Valentine's Day happened three weeks after we started dating. I remember spending the day standing in a Walgreens aisle trying to find the perfect card among the sea of pink and red flowery worded cards. I did not want to get anything overly romantic nor did I want to seem like I did not care. The pink bow with the words "Sweetheart you" around the bear's neck was an indicator that he probably had the same experience. My mind kept going back to the test. I knew what the result would be. I did not want to deal with the fact of actually knowing. I couldn't be. If I was, what was I going to do? I was over 1,000 miles away from my fiancé and the rest of my family, getting ready to move in with Kim, and still being supported by my parents. I was in no way or form ready for the responsibility that was sure to come.

The next day I woke up and found myself standing in a Walgreens aisle trying to make another difficult decision. Was it really necessary to have so many test choices? Which one should I chose: brand name or generic, digital or regular strip, most expensive or the bargain price? I swear it seemed like the universe's way to play a cruel joke on my already mentally-tortured mind. After standing in the aisle for over half an hour weighing the pros and cons of each test, I opted for a digital, generic, middle-priced test. It seemed like a reasonable compromise between all the choices. Not that the choice would have any bearing on the results.

I was barely inside my door when I began ripping open the test package and began reading the directions. I did not think that it would be possible to mess up a simple test, but I was not taking any chances. As I read the directions I began to feel as if I had chosen the wrong test:

1. Tear open the package.

2. Place the reading stick into the applicator, make sure you hear a click.

The test required assembly. I started to ask myself was this a joke. Why would the makers of this test want to further torture me by having me complete manual labor before I could even take the test? As if I wasn't anxious enough. Following the directions, I placed the stick into the applicator, but I could not distinguish the click. Had I pushed the stick too far or not far enough? I couldn't understand why the directions were so precise. Would the test not give the accurate result if I peed on it for more than five seconds or were the time units arbitrary? I mean counting using by "one Mississippi," or "one, one thousand" was similar, but not exactly the same.

As I waited for my results with the flashing clock taunting me, I began to wonder if these tests were manufactured by women. In my mind no woman would make an assembly-required test, nor would she have the result display take so long. I thought of all the ways I would tell off the test manufacturers, and direction writers, as if it were their fault that I was in this predicament. After waiting for an agonizing minute, I slowly picked up the test and took a deep breath. There in unmistakable block letters was the word I had been avoiding for days: PREGNANT. My sigh had barely been released before my phone rang. I smiled and was glad that he knew me so well.

"Baby?" My fiancé asked in both a reassuring and inquisitive voice, making me glad that I was not going through this alone.

"Yeah . . . " I paused. "Baby." ☀

Yara Massinga is a Biomed student at Barry University pursuing her Master's degree.

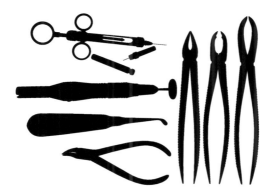

Scary Instruments

By John Holmes

Every man's fear–TURP, Transurethral Resection of the Prostate. Just the mere mention will reduce a normally healthy man to a whimpering mass of twitching flesh. Images of cystoscopes, catheters, and resectoscopes spin in their heads. To me, one of the scariest places on earth to visit is the urologist's office. There are instruments in that office for which I do not want to know their names or their purposes. I am relieved and grateful when none of the medieval accoutrements are visible during my routine visits.

Fifteen years ago, I suddenly started to feel sharp pains in my abdomen followed by urinary bleeding. I visited the urologist's office and was introduced to the cystoscope. I must have been the youngest man there by at least two decades. Not a smile in a crowd, even Don Rickels would have difficulty cracking this crowd up. The evaluation revealed an infection. I had waited much too long for treatment. The doctor explained that the infection could be cured, but more urinary problems could follow.

One year later, I had more urinary issues which required a return visit to the doctor. I was then told I had a condition called Benign Prostatic Hyperplasia (BHP) commonly called an enlarged prostate. The good news was that there was no indication of cancer, only the growing prostate. I was given a prescription and told I should be okay as long as I stayed on the meds.

The condition remained in a controlled status as long as I took my meds as required. There were times it seemed the meds were not needed and I would skip them to save money, but it did not take long for my body to remind me I needed to continue the regimen. After a period of time, the meds were less effective and a change was required. These changes seemed to coordinate with the release of newer versions of meds. The result was there never was a cheaper generic version of the prescription available to me.

My condition seemed to be controlled until about two years ago when I started to have frequent urinary urgency. I had to always know where a restroom was so if the urge struck, there would be someplace to immediately relieve myself. I went more often and was unable to pass much water. Recently, my wife and I were on vacation when the urge happened and there was no place to go. I could only sit in the car and wet into several rags in an effort to save the seat.

After that vacation, I returned to the urologist where he told me stuff I did not want to hear. There were no more meds to try and no other alternatives to control my condition except surgery. I was numb fearing what I had just heard. I envisioned the horror stories of men who had the same procedures done that my doctor had just explained to me. This was no laughing matter. Surgery of this kind could be a life changing experience.

My wife and I went home from the doctor's office and started talking about what our choices were. It seemed that there was no choice, but to have the TURP procedure done. The world seemed to spin out of sync. There was no control over the situation, only reaction to the dilemma. I called the urologist's office to set up an appointment for a final evaluation and consideration of all alternatives in preparation for possible surgery. My world got a little quieter. My enthusiasm suffered as I focused on my problem.

The doctor was prompt and the evaluation produced no additional information. My condition was stable, but would not stay that way forever. There was also the possibility of bladder problems if I waited too long. The decision was made and surgery was scheduled for the end of October.

My wife planned for us to stay at a motel the night before the procedure. We arrived on time and I was taken to the pre-op area. The staff prepared me and confirmed all of my info. For some reason, I do not think anyone would try to sneak in to where I was going. I finally was able to talk to the doctor. He explained the procedure, reiterated what was going to happen to me and the expected outcome would be. The anesthesiologist gave me options.

I interrupted him, "Just put me out." But he kept on talking.

The urologist butted in, "He just wants to go to sleep." And that was that.

The anesthesiologist went away for a brief moment and returned with a hypodermic needle. As he injected me, he stated, "This will help you relax."

Suddenly, I was aware I was being jostled on my bed. The surgery was over. I was being moved to my room for recovery. It was just like a movie with all the people in the hall moving aside as I watched the ceiling tiles rush past interrupted by florescent lights. In the room, my bed was surrounded by staff all intertwined in the collection of hanging bags, tubing, wires and blinking machines that were now my world.

Time passed quickly because of the meds. I watched the nurses and doctors go about their business of getting me back on my feet and back home. I stayed in the hospital for two days, and then the decision was made for me to be discharged to go home.

The staff disconnected much of the equipment until the time came to remove one of those scary things that urologists use. It was the drain for the surgery, very similar to a catheter. What really had me concerned was the person removing the instrument was a nursing student and had never performed this procedure before. He told me to take a deep breath and before I filled my lungs it was out. The nurse standing next to the student said she could see the color returning to my face. Boy was I relieved.

My recovery was textbook, and I improved over the next few weeks. Now when I hear stories about the urologist, I know that in the hands of experienced, competent professionals, and even young trainees, all those scary instruments can be used to heal. ☀

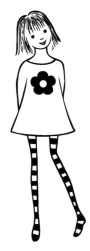

The Perfect Girl

By Gloria Lee

As she sat in her room surrounded by her numerous trophies and ribbons, Claire flipped through old pictures and started to reminisce about how she got to this point in her life.

From the day she was born, great things were expected of Claire. Her mother had gone through several rounds of in vitro fertilization to conceive her, and so the day that Claire finally arrived was nothing short of a miracle. Being the only child, she was always the center of attention. Her mother lived vicariously through her. She enrolled Claire in every extracurricular activity possible. Claire was a natural and excelled in everything she did. Her parents were always proud of her.

Every chance they got they would brag to their friends saying, "My daughter is the best. Not only does she excel in her academics, but she is also the youngest girl ever in point ballet class. Her piano teacher calls her a child prodigy!"

None of this really bothered Claire until she attended high school. The pressure to be perfect had been building up like a balloon about to burst. Her days were filled with school, followed by hours of dance, tennis and piano. She would be so occupied with her days that she soon started to skip meals unintentionally. As a result she lost a few pounds.

Her mother noticed and would compliment her saying, "Claire, you are so beautiful. You are finally getting rid of that baby fat of yours!"

These comments drove Claire to begin monitoring everything that came in contact with her mouth. She started to second guess if she was truly hungry even though her stomach growled. Claire started to consume less and less food. Some days she would only eat a handful of popcorn. On the days she did eat an entire meal, she would feel the guilt kicking in and would rush to the bathroom to regurgitate what she had just consumed.

This soon became a habit that was uncontrollable, but in Claire's eyes she felt that the only thing she had control of was her weight. Her mother controlled the other aspects in her life.

As her body started to diminish, the spirit of the girl who once had it all also started to die. Her once glowing face was now re-placed with sunken eyes and a dull complexion.

As she sat in her room, a million questions flooded her head. "How did I get to this point? What will my parents think? How can I tell them I have a problem? Will things ever go back to normal?" Although she knew this would be the hardest thing she has ever had to do, she knew that this would be the beginning to putting her life back on the right track. ☼

Gloria Lee is a graduate student in the Master of Science Program in Health Services Administration. at Barry University, Miami Shores, Florida.

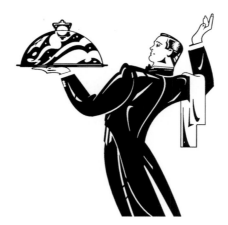

Don't I Recognize You?

By Phil Reichert

I n my new job I simply don't encounter the colorful characters I used to meet every day talking to people about their sexually transmitted diseases.

On a pleasant fall Saturday evening on St. Petersburg Beach, a mild gulf breeze blew across the parking lot as my wife, our best friends and I strolled into the Brown Derby for dinner.

A handsome, well-groomed waiter came to our table to take drink orders. The graphic on his apron stated, *BROWN DERBY, Where Interesting People Come to Dine.* His name tag said Brad.

Brad took several looks at me while he was taking our drink order. I was used to that. Gay men came into the clinic every day, and occasionally I was asked if my sexual proclivities swung in their direction. I could tell Brad wanted to ask me something when he said, "You look familiar. Have we met?"

"No, I don't think so," I replied. I recognized Brad. In the interest of confidentiality and not wishing to embarrass him, I acted as if I'd never seen him.

Let me tell you a little about my job at that time. When I wasn't having the occasional night out with my wife and friends, my job title was "venereal disease investigator," and I worked at the county health department. What I did from Monday through Friday was talk to patients who attended the VD clinic about how not to become reinfected once they were treated. I tried to figure out who infected them and who they may have infected. Then, I went into the field to find their sexual partners and get them tested and treated. My job required the utmost in confidentiality. To maintain client privacy, we could never tell a client the name of the person who provided their name. The message was generic: "An urgent matter concerning your health has come to the attention of the health department, and you may need to have tests done. You may also need medication as a preventive measure."

At the Brown Derby, my wife and friends were aware of what I did for a living. In fact, Brad wasn't the first person to recognize me from "somewhere," when they weren't sure from where. One time, I was shopping at Maas Brothers and a pretty sales clerk with neat brown hair pulled into a ponytail approached me and, before I could ask her directions to Men's Wear, she stared straight into my eyes and said, "Haven't we met?" If my wife had been with me, she would have thought the clerk was flirting with me. Quietly, I pulled the clerk aside and told her how she knew me. Then I asked her to point me in the direction of men's shirts.

With his neatly coiffed blond hair, his high cheek bones and his piercing blue eyes, Brad returned to the table with our drinks. His skin was tanned, and he was neat in the sense he might have been an actor when he wasn't making ends meet by waiting tables. Brad's delicate appearance would have made for an attractive woman. This observation came from the flaming heterosexual I was (and still am—uh, not that there's anything wrong with that). He continued to stare, and went on, "Now, I know I recognize you. Do you take classes at St. Pete Junior College?"

"No."

"Have you ever been to the Wedgewood?"

"Nope."

"Do you ever hang out at Barney's Bistro?"

"No, again."

"I know, you work at Maas Brothers." That was a little ironic, since the incident with the attractive brunette sales clerk had just taken place the week before.

I told Brad, "Sorry, no. Since I grew my beard, I've been accused of resembling Steven Spielberg, but I'm not him."

With a disappointed look, he said, "You do kind of favor Spielberg, now that you mention it. So, are we ready to order?" We told him on what we wished to dine, since we were interesting people. We embraced the slogan on his apron.

Brad returned to the kitchen to put in our order. I excused myself from the table to wash up. I found Brad, pulled him aside. In a hushed tone, I told him why he recognized me. A sudden look of terror came over his face, but just as quickly he relaxed into an "I knew I recognized you!" mode. After a thoughtful pause, Brad said, "Wow! I am glad you didn't say anything in front of your friends."

I asked, "Everything okay? No bad reactions to the penicillin injections?"

He said, "No, thanks for caring, and for the discretion."

We shook hands and I returned to the table. I sat back down to an excellent dining experience. Brad earned his tip, but was considerably less talkative as the evening progressed.

Later, when we were home alone, my wife said, "So, how did Brad take it when you told him how you knew him?" I knew she didn't expect an answer, so I just smiled. ☼

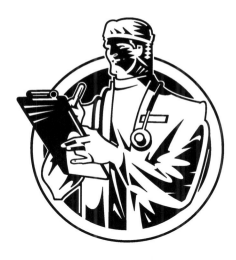

Flying into the Sun

By Rolando Garcia-Rojas

It was seven in the morning and the coffee pot was bone dry. I emptied the liquid soap into a small saucer and mixed in warm water to produce lather. I folded my lab coat neatly unto a wooden chair that served as a makeshift coat hanger for everyone in the small office.

At the Red Cross everything was donated, even the space. I chose to stay overnight because I lived in the city. Taking the bus in the morning required a 4:00 AM wake-up call. Rural clinics were the farthest from school, but the best places to learn. Unluckily, the neighbors' roosters had the alarm set for 4:15, 4:30, and 4:45 am. Falling out of bed all three times did little for my R.E.M. cycle. I could still taste the earth on my lips from the first fall.

I washed my hands as I sang "las mañanitas (the birthday song in Spanish)," finishing with my face. I combed my hair, parting to the side for added conservative professionalism, shined my clinic white shoes, and clipped the name tag on to my lapel. I put my stethoscope in my lab coat pocket and grabbed a thermometer. I quickly placed it inside my pocket as Irma, the head nurse, scolded me like a grade school principal would do for being late.

I walked up to the observation room and rubbed my shoes against the sticky, disposable floor mat. The door opened and I ran straight to the front of the providers' line. Today was the first day of clinics and I wasn't about to be left behind.

As time passed, my eyes began to itch. I rubbed a cloth over my glasses to wipe away the film of fingerprints collected over the course of twelve hours. I raised my head away from the clipboard and stared at the miniscule, square window above me in the second floor examination room. The sun came in as if to remind me the day was not over yet. It cast a beam over the corner of the desk, and I found myself inside it, lost in thought.

Listing the day's encounters, I felt like an accountant, "Eight upper respiratory tract infections, four inner ear infections, one pap smear, three elderly conversations..." The late afternoon was finally here.

I set my clipboard on the desk and inspected the last patient's historical note for errors, omissions and to fix the doodles I call handwriting. At that moment the sound of wood creaking caught my attention. It grew louder. I could see the top of a man's head making its way up the stairs. It was slightly balding with liver spots marking the skin. Slowly, the head lurched up the stairs. There weren't too many steps, but the man could have been climbing the Empire State Building in his mind. The last step was the most difficult so I rose and offered my left forearm. The dry skin of his fingertips bit into my soft skin. I pulled him up, over the last step. He pointed his chin up towards me and I could see his bloodshot, glassy eyes hemorrhaging sad memories.

"Gracias, joven," (Thank you, young man), was all he uttered, more than enough to smell day old coffee mixed with tequila.

Irma flew up the stairs and yelled, "Salte, viejo borracho!" (Leave you drunken old man!)

The man winked at me and made his way towards the chair. The head nurse proceeded to list the number of times this man had come to the clinic wasted drunk and emphatically noted his skill at harassing female attendants. I lowered my right hand and fanned outward giving her thanks, showing I was not uncomfortable with his presence. She ignored me, just staring daggers at this golem of a man as she walked down the steps, never turning her back.

I grabbed my clipboard to prepare the last patient's history of the day. I began with his name, Oracio, and skipped over the box titled "profession." Feeling him staring at me, I continued to ask him questions of age and place of residence while focusing on the paper. I sat up to finish the interview. It was at that moment that all was revealed to me.

A large belly protruded from a short-sleeved, light blue dress shirt. I could not help, but stare at this oddly, smooth hairless skin balloon. It was whiter than normal, and the veins wanted to burst all at once. It was the first person I had ever seen with advanced cirrhosis naturally brought about from years of alcohol abuse.

He asked for my name and I answered callously and dismissively. I began by asking him when he began drinking. He answered gently, "El dia que ella murio," (the day she died). Before I could ask who "she" was he uttered one name, "Sofia," and he painted with words the most beautifully, tragic picture I had ever heard.

Sofia had been a law student at the city university where Oracio studied engineering. They met in the lobby of the faculty building shared by both departments, a casual run-in consisting of a bump and the dropping of papers followed by apologies and smiles. He confessed the accidental meeting had been planned days before after seeing her. Oracio swore to himself he would talk to her even if she dismissed him. The story was a tornado, her eyes, her love, his heart and devotion. They married before graduation and bliss granted both wings for five long years.

It was at the end of the fifth year, Sofia discovered she could not bear children. He was devastated at the thought, no possibility of a family with his beautiful love. Still he knew her pain was greater than his. She faulted herself daily, tormenting, flagellating with words and feelings of despair. He tried to comfort her many times only to see her pull away like an injured bird, flightless and in pain. His pain turned to anger. How could she have pushed him away after their ordeal, he wondered. He was angry at her, angry at her ego. She could only see her pain, no room for his love.

Up to this point, Oracio's eyes were red and watery but I assumed it was from the high blood pressure, a symptom of his failing liver. It was then that he began to gently weep. His chin fell forward and came to rest at the base of his hands, cupped together. As he spoke, Oracio, began to tremble, and I offered him some water. He dug into his left back pocket pulled out a metal flask wrapped in weathered and torn leather. Taking a swig, the yellowish liquid ran down the side of his cracked lower lip. I could smell the aged tequila and closed my eyes as I pinched my nose.

"Es para curar los huesos," (this is to heal the bones), he muttered.

I could tell he had more courage now. I asked him if his wife would approve of his drinking.

Oracio closed the flask and whispered, "Los muertos no tienen opinion," (the dead don't have an opinion). He proceeded to tell me how she was making her way back home one day from clerking with a law firm, standing at the bus stop forgetting the day's affairs, sipping on an ice coffee. He said Sofia was still in pain but a few days before she mentioned a dream that struck him as strange, different than what she had been feeling. In the dream, Sofia said, she and Oracio were flying and happy. She let go for one instant and happiness filled her soul. In her dream she turned to Oracio and smiled, but he was far away still flying with her just no longer at her side. She was consumed with happiness and continued to fly as he drifted farther away. I could tell this bothered him, her happiness and the thought of his isolation. Then she mentioned he vanished, only to reappear next to her. Hand in hand they flew into the sun, laughing.

I asked him if he knew what the dream meant. He brushed aside my psychoanalysis. He stood up with more energy than when he arrived and asked, "Te gusta quien eres, tu tienes un amor?" (do you like who you are, do you have a love?). Before I could answer he told me Sofia was struck and killed by the bus that she waited for on that street corner. He mentioned how strange it was that she would be so distracted as to not see such a big bus coming at her on that particularly long street. I shook my head in disbelief and asked why she was distracted.

Oracio quickly answered, "Ya estaba volando," (she was already flying).

He asked me once more if I had a love. I half answered that I had just broken up with my girlfriend of three years. I told him of our plans to marry and how that was no longer an option.

He said, "Con amor siempre hay solucion," (with love there is always a solution).

Oracio now began to make his way to the stairs and thanked me for my time. I noticed that the sun no longer cast itself on the chair, but a sliver of light cut the floor sideways. I asked if he knew the meaning of his name.

He answered affirmatively, "Latin, significa tiempo," (Latin, it means time) and slowly made his way down into the waiting area below.

I heard a week later from Irma, the head nurse, Oracio was found dead in his home. Like most alcoholics with cirrhosis, he asphyxiated on his own vomit and blood. Still I remember our chat that afternoon and the burden of pain he shared with me. I always wondered if he knew the name Sofia comes from the Greek meaning wisdom. I was wiser after that day about life, love and time. ☼

Rolando Garcia-Rojas is a graduate of the University of Miami, FL focusing on Microbiology and Immunology. Mr. Garcia-Rojas studied medicine at the Autonomous University of Guadalajara in Jalisco, Mexico and is currently enrolled in the dual master's program for Health Services Administration and Public Health at Barry University. Mr. Garcia-Rojas currently works as a clinical research coordinator for the South Florida VA Foundation for Research and Education at the Miami VA Hospital with a focus on Hepatitis C.

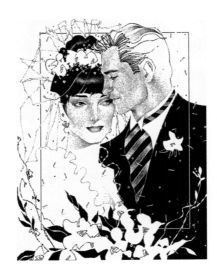

A Time for Every Purpose

By Megan Madge

"Mom, I had a dream that I became a nun!" Megan said through laughter, her voice still scratchy. "What if I'm forced to become a nun? I swear all of the boys at Michigan State have actually regressed in age. You should have seen them during Halloween last weekend! A few fraternity guys actually wore little girl's Disney princess costumes."

Bree chuckled and paused from making the bed. "And you wonder why you've gone through four years of college and haven't met anyone you're remotely interested in? Well don't worry honey, it's just not time yet. The Bible says, "To every thing there is a season, and a time to every purpose under heaven," she said. Bree's aqua eyes sparkled, as she continued, "Meg, like I said last night, you're only a senior in college. You're not supposed to have it all figured out just yet. That's what this stage of your life is all about honey."

Meg looked perplexed. The unexpected always made her uneasy. She persisted, "But Mom, you've been with Dad for 35 years, so that would have made you 16 when you met. I'm 22 and I don't think I'll ever meet someone that I will want to be with forever. How did you know?"

"You just will," Bree responded as she placed pillows on the bed. "But how, Mom?" Megan whined jokingly. Bree looked at her daughter with a laugh and said, "Okay put it this way. Whoever that person is must be someone that you will be happy with even under the worst circumstances. Look at your dad and me. If I didn't truly love him, taking care of him all these years in poor health wouldn't have been possible for me. But our life together is full of joy, even despite the rough patches with his health. Our relationship is based on a genuine friendship, common values and respect. Not anything superficial. And...we laugh a lot, which definitely helps."

Megan parsed her lips and paused to process this advice. "Okay that makes perfect sense. So, if I could be happy with someone even under bad circumstances like an illness that would be a sign?"

"Exactly," Bree nodded.

Three years later, Megan sat hunched over with her arms crossed, her right leg shaking incessantly. She watched vigilantly at every person that walked past the cracked door, hoping it was the doctor. The wait was killing her.

Without realizing it, her mind traveled to the past. She remembered lying under the Cancun sun on her honeymoon just months before, and she remembered the day when her husband Joe, a thirty-year-old Naval officer, left for Iraq. Megan thought to herself, "It's understandable to expect your first year of marriage to be the toughest. But how is it possible that we spend the first four months with Joe in Iraq, and then when he finally comes home he gets diagnosed with cancer? Well, it can't get worse than this." The previous year provided her with major perspective on what an actual "crisis" was. She marveled at how unexpected life could be.

Joe's warm, strong hand on her neck quickly brought her mind back to the present. He whispered, "I'm sure everything is okay, Honey. Please don't worry." Megan looked up at his kind brown eyes and tried to form a smile. It still amazed her every time he was the one comforting her. The man next to her looked like a shell of the tall, dark and handsome man she married. But his calm and collected attitude was always consistent. Joe's usual 6'1" muscular frame had turned frail and weak. His normal tan complexion looked gray and ghostly. His head was bald. His eyebrows were scarce. And, his eyelashes left no trace. She put her focus back on his warm brown eyes and nodded.

"Have you called your Mom yet?" Joe asked. Megan stared lifelessly at the gray tile floor and silently shook her head. "I just don't want to dampen her spirits. Mom is probably doing some last-minute things for my sister's wedding. And...I really don't want to leave you here waiting alone."

"I'm fine," he said strongly. Megan stood up reluctantly. "Honey, look at me," Joe said seriously. "No matter what the tests say, you have to get on that plane tomorrow morning and go home for your sister's wedding. I can stay in the hospital if need be. You can't miss being your sister's maid of honor." The intense mental training Joe had received in his career taught him to handle challenging situations with ease, but this time was different. It concerned her that he needed to be so independent.

Megan reflected on that morning's events. It was the first time Joe ever really looked scared. He was coughing up blood, which meant the chemotherapy drugs may have damaged his lungs permanently. Joe always believed he could defeat cancer, but losing his lung capacity meant also losing his career. This undoubtedly terrified him. Without passing the strenuous military physical fitness tests, his life would be permanently scarred. There would be no way to wake up from this nightmare.

Lung damage would also mean that Joe's last round of chemo, scheduled for the following week, would have to be postponed. He would have no choice, but to repeat treatment from the beginning. Those drugs, which are needed to sustain him throughout treatment, caused horrendous side effects. Megan couldn't bear the thought of seeing her husband suffer all over again, but what else could they do? Her worry weighed her heart down.

She approached a window outside the cancer floor, checked her phone for a signal, and with her heart racing, made the call.

"Hi Meg!" Her Mom answered in one ring. "I'm with your sister picking up her wedding dress. She looks..."

Megan interrupted her. Tears ran down her face as she spoke, "We're back at the hospital. Joe's coughing up blood, a lot of blood. I wanted to call you because I promised not to hold anything back. I don't think I can come in for the wedding at this point. I just can't leave him. He may have to start treatment all over again."

"Oh Megan! Don't worry about your sister. She understands that you must focus on Joe. I wish I could be there, Honey. I'm so sorry. I love you."

As she walked back to the room to see Joe, Megan remembered her mother's words: "Whoever that person is must be someone that you will be happy with even under the worst circumstances." She took solace in knowing that despite whatever news they were told today, she was with "that person."

So with a sense of gratitude and faith, Megan approached Joe's room with her eyes dried and with a more courageous heart. "I need to be strong for him," she thought. "It's all about him."

The doctor's gentle knock instantly bolted the couple back into the present situation, like jumping into a pool of icy water. Immediately, Megan's chest tightened. Her heart was banging with anticipation. Joe squeezed her hand as they both stood up.

A small humble smile broke through the doctor's stoic countenance. "Sorry for the wait. Let's take a look at your MRI." Megan and Joe nodded silently.

A foggy MRI image of Joe's lungs appeared on the computer screen. Megan gasped!

"They're crystal clear!" Megan yelped with exhilaration. "Does that mean he is okay?" Megan asked excitably, ready to jump out of her skin.

The doctor spun his chair around and smiled. "Yes Mrs. Madge, he is clear as a whistle. The blood must have been from another cause, but regardless his lungs look perfect."

Joe grabbed his wife and hugged her with the same passion that he had exhibited toward her upon his return from Iraq. Megan embraced him and felt that she could explode with feelings of relief and excitement. Nothing compared to the feeling of pure joy knowing he was okay.

"I actually have even better news for you," the doctor said. "After examining the results from Joe's latest tests with the Chief of Oncology, we both agreed that the last round of chemo is unnecessary. Therefore, you are officially finished with your treatment."

Megan and Joe exchanged glances of disbelief.

"It's been a rough four months," the doctor continued. "So Joe, as long as you are up to it, I think you should go home with Megan for the wedding. You are clear to travel the distance by car. Hey, you could even drive home tonight and surprise your family."

Megan and Joe agreed with intense enthusiasm to follow the doctor's orders.

Hand in hand, the couple made their way out of the hospital. In the midst of her exhilaration, Megan recalled her mother's Ecclesiastical wisdom: "To every thing there is a season, and a time to every purpose under heaven." ✺

Megan Madge graduated from Michigan State University with a BA in Psychology. After college, she worked for a recruitment firm for five years. She is pursuing an MHSA/MPH degree due to the experience with Joe. She graduated from Barry University in the fall of 2011. Ms. Madge has been married for almost three years and her husband has been cancer free for two years!

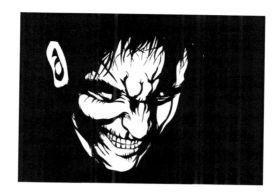

Zombie Apocalypse

By Amy Tejirian

S itting around the campfire at Bahia Honda State Park in the Florida Keys, playing UNO in the dim light, it was hard to tell the green cards from the blue ones. "Wait," my friend, Alicia, exclaimed. "I have a crank lantern we can use." She raced to the tent and snatched a big black lantern and started cranking it vigorously. "It's also a radio," she announced. After five minutes, she broke out into a sweat.

Alicia turned the light on…..only there was no light. Well, there was a glow, but definitely no useful light. It couldn't even guide us to the washrooms let alone distinguish the color of the UNO cards. Layne, Alicia's husband, and I started laughing and joking about the light, or lack thereof which quickly turned into popular light bulb jokes.

"How many journalists does it take to change a light bulb?" I quipped.

"We just report the facts, we don't change'em," Layne answered.

"Oh yeah," Alicia joined in, "How many lawyers does it take to change a light bulb?"

I answered, "You won't find an attorney who can change a light bulb. Now, if you're looking for one to screw a light bulb…"

After a good few more rounds of famous light bulb jokes, we

turned our attention back to the UNO game, but we still couldn't decipher the blue from the green cards.

"At least make that lantern useful while we play. Turn on the radio," Layne suggested.

The radio consisted of one button on the side of the giant, useless monstrosity that called itself a lantern. Alicia pressed the button trying to find a radio station. She continued pushing it, but all we could hear was static. Maybe it was because we were out in the middle of the Keys that we did not find any stations. Maybe it was because the radio was just as ineffective as the light. Layne and I decided on the latter and started making fun of it again.

"Hey, if there was a zombie apocalypse, you would all come begging to use this crank lantern," Alicia defended. "There'd be no electricity or batteries. What would you do then? This light and radio may be your only resource. Laugh now, but who'll be laughing during the zombie apocalypse."

"That lantern holds special powers to fight off zombies. Only IT can save us!" I proclaimed in a sarcastic voice.

We forgot our UNO match and started discussing the zombie uprising in great length. Layne described how he would physically fend off the attacking undead. Alicia explained how she wanted to go to a small, uninhabited key, grow veggies and live off the grid. I swore that the lantern would defend me because it must have secret powers. Or if it didn't, I could swing it at zombies to knock them out, as it was very bulky, and the protruding crank could do serious damage. Oh the joys of camping! There were no distractions like TV or Internet so good friends could enjoy each other's company and banter.

Several weeks later, I had completely forgotten about the zombie uprising chat and I went to visit my sister in New Orleans. I asked if she had any good ideas as gifts for my friends besides the usual like voodoo dolls, beads and hot sauce. Without me ever sharing my camping story with her, she recommended, "I got my friends a St. Michael medallion. He is an archangel and protects you from evil so the medal can help shield you during a zombie apocalypse. You can get them at the St. Louis Cathedral at Jackson Square. Just don't mention to them it's a safeguard from zombies."

Shocked that she too was thinking about this impending attack from the undead, I recounted my conversation with Alicia and Layne.

My sister said, "I was discussing this with my friends the other day as well, and I think that I have all the skills necessary to stave off any zombies. I'll be a commodity during the apocalypse."

"Ok, so you're a doctor and can help people medically. I give you that. But what else would make you so indispensable?"

"Your friend said she wanted to go to her own island. Can you sail a boat?...I can." She said in her best smart-alec tone.

"Ok, whatever. I'll be sure to remember when the zombie apocalypse is near."

After these two conversations, I started to hear more about this dooming event everywhere. It would frequently come up in casual conversations with other friends. Then, coincidentally, a crazy preacher named Harold Camping (that really is his last name), predicted that Judgment Day would begin on May 21, 2011. The righteous would be sent to heaven and all others left behind to suffer God's wrath. It was all over the media like a moth to a flame.

A couple days after Camping shared his prophecy, the Centers for Disease Control and Prevention published, "Social Media: Preparedness 101: Zombie Apocalypse." This guide included a brief history on zombies, (they like eating brains), and what you can do to prepare yourself in case they attack.

The first piece of advice was to have an emergency kit which, at a minimum should include:

- **Water** (1 gallon per person per day)
- **Food** (stock up on non-perishable items that you eat regularly)
- **Medications** (this includes prescription and non-prescription meds)
- **Tools and Supplies** (utility knife, duct tape, battery powered radio, etc.)
- **Sanitation and Hygiene** (household bleach, soap, towels, etc.)
- **Clothing and Bedding** (a change of clothes for each family member and blankets)
- **Important documents** (copies of your driver's license, passport, and birth certificate to name a few)
- **First Aid supplies** (although you're a goner if a zombie bites

you, you can use these supplies to treat basic cuts and lacerations that you might get during a tornado or hurricane)*

Also, the CDC suggested having an emergency plan like where to go and who to call if zombies started appearing outside your door. Again, this was also recommended for floods, earthquakes and other emergencies. The CDC assured us that if zombies started roaming the streets, they would be there to investigate and provide technical assistance, just like they do during any other disease outbreaks.

The CDC had successfully written this zombie preparedness guide to get citizens thinking and preparing for actual everyday threats. It worked. After reading this useful and reassuring information by the CDC, I felt that preparing for zombies would be like preparing for a hurricane.

According to Camping, doomsday was fast approaching. I wouldn't have to worry if I was lifted up to heaven, but what if I was left behind? What if doomsday was not as Camping described but a zombie apocalypse instead? "Maybe I should heed the CDC's advice and start getting ready," I thought to myself.

May 21 was fast approaching, yet I felt absolutely no desperation or doom. After much deliberation, I thought, "It wouldn't be SO bad to become a zombie during their apocalypse. I don't want to live the rest of my life running away from the undead and living in constant fear. Besides, I think that my friends would have tasty brains that I would enjoy feasting on." I shared these thoughts with my friends. They agreed, we all would have quite delicious brains.

"But you will be dead!" Alicia exclaimed. "You won't feel anything anymore or have any more thoughts. It won't be you."

"No, I'll be the undead." Then I started singing in my best Peter Murphy voice, "Undead. Undead. Undead."

Saturday, May 21 passed without any rapture. That worked out well since I did not bother preparing for a zombie apocalypse or any other apocalypse for that matter. "It's never going to happen to me," I kept saying.

After the media frenzy about the failed Judgment Day prediction became outplayed, the media started to focus on another threat, but this time, it was a serious, plausible one – hurricanes. Hurricane season would begin shortly, June 1. I had no supplies or plans. This was an event that could happen to me, so I considered starting to prepare, for it just as the CDC advised.

I searched and gathered my hurricane supplies that had been strewn around my apartment after last hurricane season ended – flashlights, a portable radio and Band-Aids, etc. I wrote a shopping list of other supplies I would need to restock like water, nonperishable food, and batteries. I made plans with Alicia and Layne to ride through a big storm at their place since I lived in a hurricane evacuation zone. I also marked all of the blue UNO cards so that we could distinguish them if the power were to go out and just in case my flashlight only beamed as much light as Alicia's colossal crank lantern. (Although I knew my flashlight provided much more illumination.)

Now, if zombies happened to appear in a hurricane funnel or storm surge, I would be prepared for them as well. ☼

*Centers for Disease Control and Prevention. "Social Media: Preparedness 101: Zombie Apocalypse". http://emergency.cdc.gov/socialmedia/zombies_blog.asp.

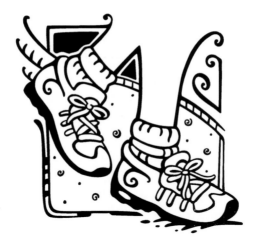

A Beautiful Obsession

By Marsha Samson

"Keep going this way and you will never find a husband!" The resonance of his voice followed me as I walked by. I could feel the fat between the thighs of my heavy frame disappoint him as I quickened my steps to walk out of his view. Like a turtle, I slouched my back to hide myself and pulled the light sweater I wore over my hands.

I started to gain weight in the ninth grade. I did not notice the added pounds or care that my clothes were becoming tighter and tighter. I did not understand the struggles that came with being hefty. America's obsession with weight loss and dieting were foreign ideas to me. And then, one day, it hit me. I was no longer one of the skinny girls. In both my eyes, and American society's, that quickly translates to no longer being attractive.

This realization made me think, "Stop eating!" but my body asked for more and my willpower was weak. I began following every fad diet in the world. I kept gaining weight. I felt powerless. I started hiding food and gaining more weight. I was ashamed, but addicted.

I tried to become a vegetarian, followed many detox plans and became self-destructive as a way to lose weight. Before the third day of every new obsession, I would quit. I continued this way for four years. Wasting hours of my day thinking of how much prettier I could be.

I went to college lacking self-esteem and doubting that I would ever find myself. I compared myself to all of the skinny girls around me. I felt uncomfortable every time I went to the gym. I sensed everyone watching me and mocking the amount of time I spent on the treadmill. I then resolved to only go to the gym if I lost ten pounds.

Needless to say, I went from -2 pounds to +10. Postponing the gym under this pretext made me gain more weight! I kept wishing that something could help me lose weight and to be beautiful again. I blamed my parents for letting me gain weight. I attributed it to my father not wanting to give me a gym membership when I was in middle school, and to my mother for letting me quit both tennis and tap dancing lessons.

Being overweight caused me to become fearful of everything weight-related. I developed gymnophobia, the fear of being nude; a gym phobia; hypothermosis, the fear of sweat-specifically sweating in public; and the fear of losing weight. Ironically, what I considered to be the root of my problems was not a solution. I began to fear that I might fail when I began the diet and this always led me to fail.

My mother sat me down and said, "You're beautiful don't waste your youth worrying about numbers on a scale." My mom just wanted me to be healthy and happy. She decided to start a diet plan with me and didn't tell anyone. I always thought that losing weight had to be this dreadful process of starvation, logging excessive hours at the gym and overall a feeling of constant dissatisfaction. My mom showed me I was wrong.

She gave me the tools to understand the importance of being healthy, which isn't necessarily skinny. Every morning she made me a blueberry or strawberry shake along with a handful of nuts. She followed it with a small salad for my first lunch and a 'green' shake for my second lunch. The 'green' shake was a mixture of dark leaves, such as kale or spinach, with celery, and either carrots or apples. At first the idea of drinking something like that completely turned me off, but, truth be told...I really grew to love the drinks. More importantly, I looked forward to the time I spent with my mom and started to realize how much she would do for me.

Throughout the day, she continued to feed me carrots, tomatoes, and for dinner would give me fish, steak, or chicken with salad and quinoa rice. I always looked forward to dessert, no matter how full I was. She varied between pineapples, watermelon, and mangoes. By the end of the diet, I wanted to change my life.

When I returned to college after a month and a half of being spoiled, I continued to take care of myself. Walking to class I felt great and confident enough to try fitness classes. I stopped feeling ugly, realizing that I am not one of those *skinny* girls, but one of those *healthy* girls.

My mother saw the beauty within me. Her faith continues to inspire me. I run three miles a week, do light weights, and maintain a healthy diet. I am now within a healthy BMI.

My mom always said *"You are as beautiful as you feel!"*

Today, I feel beautiful. ☀

Marsha Samson is a graduate student at Barry University.

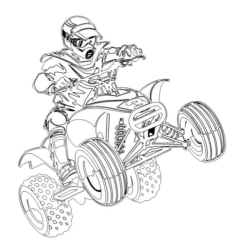

Grandma's Words

By Komarvoski Wells

The sun baked the red clay in the foothills of South Georgia as I continued my adventurous and sometimes reckless drive on my high-performance all-terrain vehicle (ATV). Riding my ATV throughout the countryside was one of the activities that signaled the end of the long, boring school year. The summer in South Georgia was the laid-back time of year when boys and girls reveled in activities that are typical of rural south Georgia, like fishing, camping, working the tobacco fields, and most of all, skinny dipping.

Like most young children of the South, my grandparents played an important role in my upbringing. Specifically, it was my maternal grandmother, Rosa Mae Wells that was the guiding force in my life. Rosa was the mother of eight children and over forty grandchildren and great-grandchildren. The granddaughter of a slave, Rosa had the character and personality that radiated compassion, hope, resilience, and wisdom. It was during the summer months that Grandma Rosa would invite the grandkids to her home in rural Georgia for rest and relaxation.

Although Grandma Rosa encouraged us kids to have lots of fun, she always spoke words of wisdom to enforce our respect for safety. However, sometimes I suppressed Grandma's words in lieu of the exhilaration that comes with racing an ATV through the winding dirt roads of South Georgia.

Of all the great summer activities for a kid to do in Georgia, riding my ATV was by far my favorite—and the most dangerous. My uncle introduced me to the world of ATVs at an early age. His voice resonated, "You must always wear a helmet, never speed, and certainly never 'hot dog.'" Of course, I reassured him that I would follow these rules. Nevertheless, my rebellious attitude flowed through me as I raced up and down the dirt roads without wearing a helmet or shirt.

Grandma also preached, "Grandson, I don't want to ever see you riding that machine without a helmet on your head and a shirt on your back!" But on that scorcher of a July afternoon, riding helmetless and shirtless, my heart rate increased, my blood vessels constricted, and my air passages dilated as adrenaline flowed throughout my body. Subconsciously, the voice of Grandma Rosa was ringing in my ears, "Grandson, you have to be sensible and always wear a helmet when you ride that doggone ATV! That thing is gonna kill you! Mark my words: It's not what you do, it's how you do it!" Her words were a premonition that was about to play out.

As I careened around what I perceived as a not-so-sharp curve, my left foot slipped off the foot peg of my ATV, and my leg became prey to the machine's knobby tires. In a split second, I could feel and hear the skin of my left calf being peeled away. I momentarily lost consciousness, waking up with the distinct smell of flesh, blood, motor oil, and hot Georgia red dirt. Fortunately for me, my cousin was pacing behind me on his ATV and went to seek assistance. All I could think of was how disappointed and angry Grandma Rosa would be once she learned of my careless accident.

My grandmother arrived and whisked me to the only emergency room within a thirty-mile radius of our rural community, where I received the care I needed.

My diagnosis was a severe laceration of my lower left leg that required a minor skin graft and lots of painkillers. Grandma Rosa showed her contempt for my poor decision. She looked me in the eye and said, "Didn't I tell you 'It's not what you do, it's how you do it?'" Then, she obeyed her words by showing me the compassion that made her the loving woman she was. After this trauma, I continued to ride ATVs and even graduated to racing in motocross on two-wheelers.

Grandma Rosa died on December 29, 1987, at the young age of sixty-seven and after a lengthy fight with lung cancer. Her untimely loss was devastating to all that loved her and were lucky enough to hear her words of wisdom and sense of compassion. To this day, Grandma's words soothe and guide me as I continue the adventurous journey of my life. Grandma's words will be with me always.

"It's not what you do, it's how you do it."

— Grandma Rosa Mae Wells (1921-1987) ☀

Komarvoski Wells is a MBA graduate student at Barry University and holds a BA in International Relations from Florida International University.

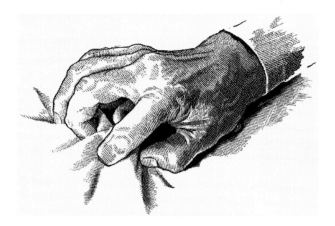

Gnarled

By Mort Laitner

I stood in front of the Barnes & Noble magazine rack wondering, "Am I in the belly of a dying dinosaur? Was this chain cruising down on the eight track highway? Better enjoy this pleasure now---it may not be around for long."

Placing my hands in my pockets, I continued reading the titles of the publications. My ring finger then tapped against my keys.

"OUCH! Damn it!" I immediately knew what was about to happen. Within a second, a sharp pain would run from my hand into the crevices of my brain. I shut my eyes as a grimace spread across my face. I could not shout nor curse in this public venue. As the pain subsided, my brain commanded, "Idiot, stop putting your hands in your pockets! You can prevent this agony. Don't touch metal."

I encountered my first arthritic trauma a year earlier. A tap on a piece of metal produced the throbbing, traveling ache. I thought, "So this is what the elderly complained about. Betty Davis had it right, 'Old age ain't for sissies.'" I now realized why senior citizens sat on their hands and declined applauding outstanding performances at Miami Beach's Jackie Gleason Theater.

I remembered gently shaking arthritic hands knowing my firm handshake could cause pain. I could now relate.

After a month of this metal-causing pain, it now occurred when I tapped on any object. My concern grew as the pain increased. In my frustration, I cursed aloud while throwing the object I held in my hand.

A few months later, I no longer had to touch anything, The pain just manifested itself out of thin air. While I tried to sleep, the throbbing kept me awake. I got up, swallowed two aspirins and eventually the pain dissipated.

A year later, I noticed a slight curvature of my left pinkie. Looking at that bent digit, I returned to glancing at the covers of the shelved magazines. One title caught my eye, —*Arthritis Today*.

I picked it up with caution as if touching it would cause all my fingers to curl.

I thought about four questions:

1. How many magazines does Barnes & Noble carry with the name of chronic diseases?
2. What is this disease all about?
3. How many Americans have arthritis?
4. Is aspirin the only palliative for my problem?

The first question was answered in a minute of magazine rack surveillance:

Two. Autism and Arthritis.

The second question was addressed throughout the magazine:

Arthritis is the wearing out of a joint, but includes more than "100" different diseases that cause pain, stiffness, swelling, and damage to the joints.

There are four main forms of arthritis:

Osteoarthritis---caused by wear, tear and trauma to the joints.

Rheumatoid arthritis---an autoimmune disease.

Gout—caused by too much uric acid accumulating in the blood.

Pseudo gout—is the result of too much calcium building up in joints.

The causes for most forms of arthritis are not known.

Sub-question: Which of the 100 arthritic diseases do I have?

Sub-answer: Time to go to the doctor to find out.

The third question was answered in the same article:

WOW. Fifty million Americans have some form of the disease. Osteoarthritis is the most common form affecting about 16 million

Americans, while rheumatoid arthritis, affects about 2.1 million and is the most crippling form of the disease.

The fourth question's answer was found on multiple pharmaceutical advertisements which filled full pages of the magazine. In fact, 50% of the mag's pages were ads for meds.

Now that I had the answers, I returned the magazine to its rightful spot on the rack. I examined my fingers--no sign of curling. I had just read Arthritis Today for free. Barnes & Noble hadn't made a dime.

I am the poison in the belly of the dinosaur. ☼

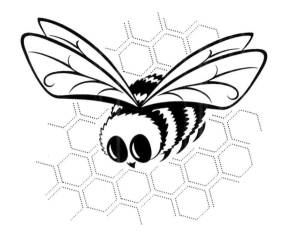

Nature's Lessons

By Jack Levine

Amidst all of the political wrangling and dizzying gyrations of the financial markets, my thoughts seek refuge in nature. I find contemplating the connections we have to the natural world gives me a needed perspective and provides me an opportunity to learn how to balance the pressures of the day.

I'll share three observations which I hope will resonate with you.

The first is an event which I believe we can all relate to....saving a creature from peril. Just the other morning I was out early to fetch the newspaper and noticed a box turtle making his way across the street. He was about the size of a large grapefruit, and moved oh so slowly across the pavement. Fearing for his safety, I approached and grabbed him by the top shell...which he did not like.

After momentarily withdrawing himself into his shell, he decided to take action and began protesting his capture by thrashing all four legs and stretching back his wrinkled neck with the intent of biting me. Not able to make contact, his final act of offense was letting forth a stream of pee, which my bare leg felt within a split second. Now it was my move. Without any duplicated act of retribution (that would have been quite a neighborhood scandal), I walked with my new pal to a wooded lot down the block ensuring his safe haven.

And off he sauntered...safe and somewhat satisfied that I learned not to mess with him.

The lesson...Some good deeds are initially rebuffed, even within our own families, but we must persevere despite the rejection in order to accomplish a necessary goal.

The second story is about our Satsuma tree, a citrus variety native to Asia which has become a North Florida favorite because of its capacity to survive an occasional cold snap. In fact, a well-timed cold snap just prior to its winter ripening makes the Satsuma fruit all the sweeter. Planted as a small sapling some eight years ago, our tree never produced any, but a small number of immature buds, which soon died and dropped. But this summer, to our great delight, our Satsuma has branched out and produced some 90-100 nice-sized fruits. Already larger than golf balls, they will surely double in size as they mature from dark green to brilliant orange by December. I find myself visiting the Satsuma nearly daily, watching with great satisfaction how a seemingly infertile tree has now become a bountiful delight.

The lesson...Sometimes nature takes its time in producing a positive outcome. Like with the developing child, full progress is not achieved by calendar alone, but by a series of experiences which we do not control, but do our best to guide to maturity.

And third...My wife and I have some 30,000 new additions to our family. We are beekeepers! As of early March, our hive has been built, stocked, and populated by a healthy colony of active (yup... busy) and productive bees. Charlotte has primary responsibility for the apiary tasks...I serve as the encouraging supporter and photographer, keeping a chronicle of the progress.

Because of bees' vital role in plant pollination, and of course their production of honey, we have been quite taken by the wonder of the process. Never before have we learned more about how a natural culture can be so smartly structured to get the job done with great efficiency.

We are now enjoying our second harvest of delicious honey... our biscuits sing its praises before succumbing to our hungry bites. We're certain that the benefit to the floral health of our neighborhood far outweighs the effort we have expended in this enterprise. In just six short months we've learned to respect the power of the honey bee for its diligence and wondrous capacity to perform its duties.

The lesson...Learning a new skill has both educational and emotional rewards. Giving nature the chance to flourish by promoting the growth of our bee colony is a sweet reminder of the connection between humans and our creature friends.

Nature's lessons can give meaning to our human struggles and provide a vital reminder that we are all linked, across the species, in our inter-dependency. ☀

Jack Levine, founder of 4Generations Institute, is a public policy advocate who lives in Tallahassee. He sends an occasional e-message to his advocate network and can be reached at jack@4Gen.org or visited at www.4Gen.org.

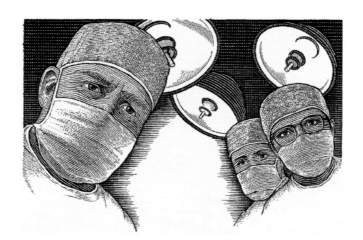

First Cut

By Clayton Jeans

As soon as the surgeon saw me, things happened fast. I was in surgery in less than 45 minutes. To put that into perspective, I had been in wincing pain for 8 hours before someone saw me, and in 45 minutes, there was already a remedy. I will never go to the ER again. They can eat it. I would sooner run full speed into a brick wall before I go to that ER again. I'll just cut myself open next time – at least it would save me some money and grief.

Anyway…so I am now under the knife.

Surgery is a strange thing. Everything seems cold and distant. I felt alone and vulnerable waiting to be wheeled into the operating room. Before, during and after surgery, you relinquish all control over your life. You put your well-being in the hands of someone you hardly know and quite possibly will never see again. You get laid out on a table and exposed physically and emotionally.

I do not like being exposed emotionally.

This is one of the things I have tried to overcome throughout this experience. This is just one of the things which are unavoidable in life sometimes. The doctors and nurses can see the fear in your eyes as they walk around you. They can feel the anxiety in your heart.

All of these feelings rush into you until... darkness. The anesthesia hits.

The appendectomy was a very routine surgery. No complications, nothing more than a two-day visit to the hospital. Other than a little soreness and a lot of animosity towards the emergency room, I was back on my feet in no time.

And showing off my scar to boot!

The following week I was to go back to see Doctor Ratliff for the removal of my stitches and for a medical rehash of the procedure. It was there that the wheels came completely off the bus.

January 20, 2005.

He gave me a quick explanation of the procedure as he was taking the stitches out. I was happy to have them removed and ready to get back to the swing of things. However, I wasn't anywhere near prepared to hear or even understand what he was about to tell me.

His demeanor should have given it away that he was about to tell me something rather unpleasant, but I just wasn't clicking on all cylinders this day. With a look of guilt stricken regret about him, he informed me that pathology found a tumor in their examination of the appendix, which was the cause of the appendicitis.

Did you say tumor? As in cancer?

The cancerous tumor was discovered in the post-operation pathology exam. Dr. Ratliff didn't even know until a week after the surgery. So there I am, after two days in the hospital and into my first week of recovery, thinking I was just another victim of a useless organ causing trouble. Not so.

I tried to convince myself and the Doc that this could in fact not be true by exclaiming in my best Arnold Schwarzenegger voice, "It's not a tumor." But as we all have probably found out in life, things we desperately want are not always made to be.

Silence.

What I have discovered is that it is hard to understand anything spoken to you once you hear news like that.

I was told that another surgery called a right-hemicolectomy needed to be performed and it needed to be done as soon as possible. The purpose of the hemicolectomy is simply to remove part of the colon and surrounding lymph nodes to see if the cancer had spread.

I was numb. It felt like I was floating as I left his office. I couldn't feel my legs, arms, feet – nothing. I sat down on the floor in the hospital hallway, I don't even know for how long, and stared at the wall. I couldn't walk, and I couldn't even talk. I was just empty and shaking.

At this moment, I was terrified. All I could think about was the negative connotations of cancer. I wasn't educated like I am today. I could only visualize sickness and death. I felt powerless, as if I had no control of my body and no control of my future. I wasn't even sure I had a future any more. The only thing I knew about cancer was what I saw with my uncle.

My uncle died of throat cancer in 2000. I can remember visiting him shortly before his death. The disease had spread so far up his throat that he couldn't talk. He couldn't even breathe without a tracheotomy. I remember him lying there in his bed at home with tubes plugged into him. I remember the sound of those machines humming in the background, essentially keeping him alive. I was so scared to see him as I walked into his room. I couldn't even recognize him. The disease had completely overrun his body. I can recall him almost lighting up and smiling as I walked into the room, despite his condition. I remember immediately breaking into uncontrollable tears. They poured down my face so hard and so fast. I left the room and went outside. I couldn't bear to see him this way. This is the only knowledge I have of cancer. Pain and death.

I felt scared.

I felt weak.

I felt cheated.

I felt my life spinning out of control.

When I revisit these moments, not much changes. I still feel scared, I still feel vulnerable and I still feel numb. This is what cancer can do to you. It blinds you and cripples you.

Finally, I found the ability to call my boss, told him I wasn't going to come back to the office that day and vaguely repeated what the doctor said to me. There was a moment of silence on the other end of the phone.

I called my mother and tried to walk her through what the doctor had told me, although I do not think anything I was saying was discernable.

I cannot recall how I made it back to my house, but one of my roommates was home when I arrived. This was strange considering it was in the middle of the workweek. I walked in, poured a strong Vodka and Sprite for myself and sat down on the couch.

I popped a couple of pain pills that had been prescribed to me for my post appendectomy pain relief – certainly more than recommended dosage (not to mention I now had a stiff alcoholic drink).

His expression asked, "What the hell is wrong with you?" And, I tried again to explain what the doctor had told me. However, I'm sure it was quite difficult to understand me. This was also the guy who not much more than a week before had buried his father.

Would have been nice to have some lighthearted and entertaining news instead...

There isn't much more of the day that I can recall. Which is strange, one would think you would remember every little thing that happened on such a day. Looking back on it – it is all a big black hole to me.

Helplessness and fear is all I can bring to mind. What had seemingly been a routine everyday surgery had led to the scariest day of my life, or so I thought. Life began to speed up and spin out of control. I never want to have another day like that again. ☀

Clayton Jeans resides in Houston, TX. He received his undergraduate degree from the University of Texas and his MBA at the University of Houston. He works in the field of oil and gas.

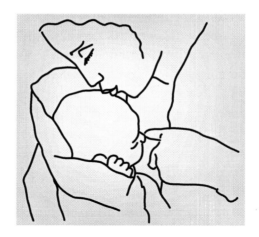

You Make
A Difference

By Ana Martinez

Dear WIC family,

Today is my last day of employment here at WIC (Women, Infant and Children), and I wanted to share my story with all of you. I couldn't leave without ensuring you all knew the difference YOU make here at WIC. Although, at times we feel overworked, over tired, under appreciated, and overwhelmed, I assure you, it is not in vain.

I was 18 years old when I first heard of the WIC program. In fact, the reason I heard of it, like many young moms, was because I was in trouble. I was young, single, fresh out of high school, scared, and, yes, pregnant. I was truly in need. Not only in need of financial assistance, but above all things, in need of sound advice and encouragement to make the right decisions for me and my unborn baby.

My first visit to WIC was in the West Perrine office where I met Mrs. Mathewson. I still remember her wearing her white lab coat every time I saw her and always being extremely patient with me every time we met for my follow-ups. She taught me about breast-feeding and encouraged me to take care of myself throughout my pregnancy. I was very interested in everything Mrs. Mathewson had to say. I nursed my son for over 10 months and I followed her advice throughout the time I saw her until my son was 2 years old. This is where my love for nutrition began! I didn't even know such a career existed. Mrs. Mathewson's encouragement and support even spurred me to enroll in school to learn more about nutrition. Once I graduated from college, I knew this is where I wanted to work. I wanted to make a difference in a young mom's life, just as Mrs. Mathewson did for me.

Now, eight years after my first day of employment at WIC and 13 years after the first day I walked in to West Perrine, I leave our program with great gratitude. I thank God for the opportunity to have made a difference & thankful for all the beautiful moms, babies, and kids I have had the pleasure of helping. WIC made a difference in me as a young mother, and my life since has been a testament to the work we do everyday.

I encourage all of you to continue giving your best each and every day, for your work does not go unnoticed. YOU make a difference!

I will miss my WIC family dearly and thank you all for all the wonderful memories.

May God continue to bless each and every one of you!

Sincerely,

Ana

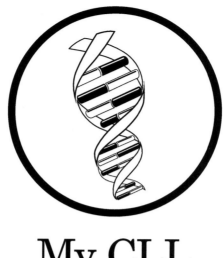

My CLL

By Avi Stavsky

"Well," said the hematologist, "all the tests point to the same diagnosis: you have CLL."

The fear at the back of my mind was thus realized. I heard his words, but did not want to believe them. Like Hosni Mubarak, I was "In D-Nile"... And yet I knew he was right, because my own mother, may she rest in peace, passed away 20 years ago from this same strange malady.

And strange indeed it is. Chronic Lymphocytic Leukemia is a type of cancer of the blood and bone marrow — the spongy tissue inside bones where blood cells are made. It is the most common type of leukemia in adults. In some people, CLL can remain slow-growing for years and may never require treatment. In others, treatment may be needed as soon as the disease is discovered.

With me, it was a routine visit to my general practitioner, who did an annual blood test. My test came back with higher than usual white blood cells. When a retest a few weeks later didn't show a drop in white blood cells, I was referred to the hematologist, who did more specialized tests as well as a CT scan. All this came less than 18 months after my successful bout against melanoma. Perhaps strangely, I took this news with more calm than I might have supposed. Maybe it's because CLL was at the back of my mind for all these years. I go to bed at night pretty much the same person I was before my diagnosis in August, 2011.

That said...something is different. While CLL is not infectious and thus people don't need to be in fear of me contaminating them, I know I cannot donate blood. I look in the mirror in the morning and see the same face. The same person, and yet...am I really?

Friends and family have reacted differently. For my wife and son, the surprise was much greater, yet they, too, remain upbeat.

"You're living in the 21st century in a country with some of the best medical care available. There are treatments and discoveries now which didn't exist when you mother first got CLL." Quite true.

Fortunately, I seem to belong to the slow and chronic rather than the acute and virulent group. The hematologist said, "You're more likely to die in a terrorist attack than by CLL." That said, the disease does need monitoring and testing every several months.

CLL runs in my family. Not only my mom, but her uncle had it too. He died in 1948 at age 78. It seems to strike Jewish families who originally came from Central and Eastern Europe.

In older adults (i.e. greater than 65), it is seldom treated by chemotherapy, which is a "cure" that can be more debilitating than the disease. However, recent clinical trials have shown that some potent fighters of this and other blood cancers are foods as mundane as green tea and turmeric, with added benefit from Vitamin C and even garlic.

Laboratory research determined that a compound in green tea extract, called EGCG, can kill CLL cells. In a study of people with early-stage Chronic Lymphocytic Leukemia, taking EGCG in pill form reduced some signs of the disease in a portion of the participants. For instance, some participants noticed that their enlarged lymph nodes decreased in size and blood tests revealed some participants had fewer leukemia cells in their blood. Research into EGCG and green tea is ongoing.

Turmeric is a common ingredient in Indian food and yellow mustard. Its active ingredient is curcumin, which gives turmeric its yellow color.

Adding curcumin to human cells with the blood cancer multiple myeloma, Dr. Bharat B. Aggarwal of the University of Texas

MD Anderson Cancer Center in Houston and his colleagues found, stopped the cells from replicating. And the cells that were left died. Although the study did not test the benefits of curcumin in patients, previous research has shown the substance may fight other types of cancers, including CLL.

Hey, that beats suffering through chemo any day, right?

As for the rest, only time will tell. I am advised to exercise regularly, to eat a nutritious diet with emphasis on green, leafy vegetables as well as the yellow and orange kind (squash, carrots, pumpkin), which are storehouses of beta-carotene.

CLL brought an emotional roller-coaster to my family, as there are so many variables and possibilities. Maybe the hardest thing to do is to plan for the long-term future. Where will I be in three years from now? In five? And will I make ten?

There are some parallels with people who found out they were HIV-Positive. Magic Johnson tested positive in 1991, yet continues to live and work almost as though it didn't affect him. He takes a combination of drugs, but otherwise goes about his business fairly normally. I see myself in somewhat the same way. Should I worry about it? And if I did...would that help?

My mother probably had CLL for several years before it was diagnosed. Again, it was discovered based on a blood test that showed abnormally high white blood cells. But for years afterward, she lived her life from day to day. If she worried, she never showed it. She had more concern for my dad, who was ten years her senior.

If I have to live with CLL, then so be it, and live is what I intend to do. And having faith in God doesn't hurt either, as I firmly believe no one goes before his time. ☼

Avi Stavsky is a retired resident of Los Angeles, California.

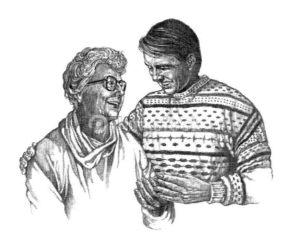

Sacrifice

By Barry R. Eisler

Today my dad passed away in his sleep at the age of 90. My mother didn't express any emotion because…she is suffering from Alzheimer's. She started developing the disease five years ago, after she turned 85. As the disease progressed and my mother's memories began to slowly erode, my father began taking more and more care of her. He did everything including bathing and feeding her.

I knew that Alzheimer's disease progresses at different rates in each person. Diagnosis to death can last from three to twenty years. There was no way to predict the life expectancy of my mother. Even though my father was also 85 and frail, he refused to allow my mother to be taken to a nursing home. He had a nurse come in once a day to assist him. I admired my dad for his selfless act.

I am an only child. I guess you could say I was spoiled. From my earliest memories, my parents, Edward and Elizabeth, always gave me everything. I remember when I was five and I wanted a pony. My dad drove me to a farm thirty miles away every weekend so I could ride. I remember whenever I was sick my mother would always stay home to take care of me. I was never in fear of being left alone because I knew that one of my parents would always return to be with me. We weren't rich. My father was a postman and my mother a waitress. However, my parents made sure I was well-fed, had nice clothes and all the latest toys and games.

As a young man graduating high school, my parents said, "We've saved up enough money to send you to a prestigious college." I didn't realize it at the time, but they had given up a lot to give me these gifts and opportunities.

As I think back, I don't recall my parents buying expensive things for themselves or going on vacations. My dad had the same two suits all his adult life and my mom sewed her own dresses.

After college I got a great job offer which if I accepted, would take me far away from home and my parents. Mom and Dad again were unselfish, and they convinced me to take the job. I knew they would miss me, but I had to start this chapter of my life.

Except for the occasional visits on holidays, living far from my parents didn't really allow me to see them much. However, we kept in touch the usual ways. Eventually they accepted my gift of a computer. They were not computer savvy, but both learned to email letters using, as my dad would say, "that new-fangled gizmo."

Now with my father gone and my mother's medical condition deteriorating, being the "only child" took on a greater significance.

I read a bumper sticker once that said, "Be nice to your kids. They'll choose your nursing home." Well now I was faced with that decision or I could follow my dad's lead and take care of my mother.

I remembered reading that 70% of people with dementia die in nursing homes. Did I want to add my mother to that statistic? Placing her in the care of someone else would have certainly been simpler than flying her 3000 miles to my home out west. I didn't even know if I was mentally equipped to be around someone who was chronically ill. I never even had a pet to care for. My life was simple. But this was my mother. She and Dad did everything for me. I couldn't turn my back on her now when she really needed me. She didn't remember any of the countless memories that touched my life, but I will carry those memories with me forever.

My mom is coming home with me. I will make the sacrifice. ❉

Barry Eisler is a retired registered respiratory therapist residing in Broward County. He is a graduate of the University of Florida, where he was a member of the Glee Club. Barry still enjoys singing and writing music.

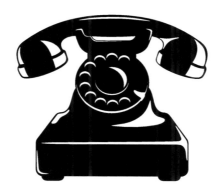

The Call

By Jennifer Douek

I t was a dreadful Sunday afternoon back in chilly November. My bags were packed as I sat quietly in my family room waiting for a phone call from my friend Rich. He was on his way to pick me up. We were heading back to Orlando after our Thanksgiving break of our first semester at the University of Central Florida. I dreaded saying goodbye to my family. Twenty minutes passed and my phone finally rang. It was Rich. My mom, dad, brother and sister, helped me carry my stuff out to the car as we said our goodbyes with tears running down our faces. I climbed in the passenger side of Rich's black BMW, rolled down the window and said, "Goodbye family, love you! I'll see you in two weeks!"

Mom said, "Don't forget to call us every hour."

"Ok mom!" I replied as we drove off.

Before I knew it, we were an hour into our trip and it was time to call home. "Hi mom, I'm calling to check in. We are still alive."

"Good! Where are you guys?" she said. "We are near Boynton Beach," I said.

Mom replied, "Ok, call in an hour."

"Will do. Love you. Bye" I said.

"Love you too." Mom said.

The second hour of traveling passed quickly and it was time for my second call. I called my house again, but no one answered. I tried again a few minutes later. Still no answer, so I called my mom's cell phone and she quickly answered. "Why didn't anyone answer at home?" I asked.

"We are just running an errand," she said.

"Ok I'll call back in an hour," I said. Rich and I talked. We were so involved in our conversation that I almost missed the three-hour mark.

I dialed home, but it went to voicemail. I called my mom's cell phone.

"Hello." My mom answered.

"Hi mom, where are you guys?" I asked.

"We are still running our errand," She said.

"OK, well we only have an hour left. We are by mile marker 185," I said.

"Drive safe, and just call my cell when you get back to your apartment." She responded.

"Ok, will do." And I hung up the phone. "Rich, it's so weird that my parents are still not home on a Sunday night."

"Don't worry Jenny. I'm sure they just had to go get some stuff."

"Ok. I guess..."

We pulled onto I-4 in Orlando and I knew we only had a half hour left. I was so excited to get out of the car.

Finally, I was back in my apartment and started to unpack. I decided to call my mom and let her know I was back safe. I dialed her cell phone. "Hi Mom, I'm back. I saw so many cops and I even saw this car crash where the car was stuck up on the metal railing in the median. It was scary."

"Well I'm glad you're back safe. Do me a favor, she said. Go stand next to your roommate Hannah."

"Okay..." I was confused as I walked over to my roommate.

"Honey... Dad had a heart attack," Mom's voice broke. I fell to the floor in shock as tears streamed down my face.

"I want to come home! I want to come home!" I screamed.

"It is too late to fly home tonight, but I will get you on the first flight home tomorrow morning!" Mom replied.

"Okay, okay... but what happened?"

"Well, about an hour after you left, dad started to grab his chest and pace around the house. I asked him if he was ok and he said that his chest hurt a little, but he thought it was just heartburn. I suggested that we go to the hospital, but he said he was fine. After about an hour he was still pacing and holding his chest. I knew something was wrong so we raced over to Baptist. I pulled up to the emergency room entrance, Jon got out of the car and helped dad in while Jackie and I went to park the car. By the time I got inside, Dad was already being wheeled away to surgery because he started to have a heart attack right there in front of everyone. Right now we are still waiting to see what is happening. I will call you as soon as I know more. Auntie Fern is booking your flight now and will e-mail you the ticket."

I could barely get any words out. "Ok" is all I could say. I sat on the floor and continued to cry. After what seemed like an eternity, I got up and started to repack my suitcase.

It was around 10:15 pm when my Mom finally called. "Dad is out of surgery. He had to have three stents put in his arteries. One was 100% blocked so they could not do anything to that one, but the other three, one was 95% blocked, another was 86% blocked and the last was 80% blocked. They have him in a medically induced coma so he doesn't wake up and become uncomfortable. As of now he is stable and the doctors said the first 24 hours are the most critical. Try to get some sleep since your flight leaves bright and early tomorrow. I will call you if anything changes. Love you."

"Love you too, Mom." I hung up the phone, jumped in the shower and then went to bed.

My alarm clock went off at 4:00 am. I slept for maybe an hour. I got dressed, loaded my stuff in Hannah's car and we were off to the Orlando International Airport. I boarded the Southwest plane for my short 30-minute flight to Miami. Scott, my boyfriend, was waiting at the airport for me. He hugged me and told me everything would be okay. He drove me home. I got in my car and rushed over to pick up my brother and sister from school. We headed over to Baptist Hospital to meet my Mom. I ran up to my Mom in tears. "Can I see Dad?"

"Not now sweetie. There are specific visiting hours in the ICU."

After five hours, they allowed me to see my father. I quietly walked down the halls of the ICU. Nervous, with knots in my stomach, I was not sure what I was about to see. I walked into my dad's room... he was on a breathing machine, lifeless. The only sounds I could hear were the beeping noises from all of the machines hooked up to him. I stood there thinking how I had just seen him the day before walking around and talking. I couldn't hold back my tears. I walked out of his room and took one more last glance at him before returning to the waiting room.

My dad was in the hospital for a week, an eternity for me. Sunday arrived and I had to go back to school. I had no desire to go back to Orlando, but I kept telling myself, "Only one week left, only one week left!" We found out that day that my dad was able to go home. We were so ecstatic and I wanted to wait to see him leave the hospital. Unfortunately, all of the paperwork and doctors took too long and I had to leave.

I sat on a chair next to my dad's bedside in silence. I was dreading saying goodbye. My mom looked at me and said, "You better get going or you will miss your flight."

I hugged each one of my family members and told them "I love you." I hugged my dad extra tight and made sure to tell him twice that I loved him. "I'll see you guys in a week," I said as I walked out of the hospital room.

"Call me when you get back to your apartment," my mom said.

"Ok, Mom. Love you."

I was on my way back to Orlando to finally finish my freshman fall semester, with tears rolling down my face. However, this time they were "happy tears."

Jennifer Douek attended the University of Central Florida and received a Bachelors Degree in Interdisciplinary Studies as well as three minors in Hospitality, Elementary Education and Criminal Justice. Currently, she is pursuing her Masters Degree at Barry University in Health Service Administration. She enjoys going to the beach, spending time with family and friends, watching movies, and traveling.

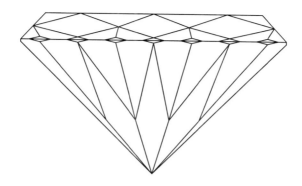

Blood Computers

By Mort Laitner

I sat behind my office desk and joyfully tapped on my new iPad 2 when a sharp burning sensation ran through my gnarled knuckles to the hidden recesses of my brain. My fingers curled and cramped as I cursed, "DAMN IT!" followed by a chorus of, "Ride the pain, ride the pain, and ride the pain." My eyes shut as I saw my hands covered in dark red blood.

As the pain subsided, I rose, opened my eyes and observed my blood-free fingers drop the iPad 2 as if it were a hot skillet.

My stomach tightened as I remembered a TV show where young Chinese workers jumped off of tall factory buildings. I closed my eyes as their bodies splattered on the good earth. Their tolerance for life ended because they worked—ten to fourteen-hour days—six days a week. Repetitively, they inserted computer chips in electronic devises, such as my iPad 2. In factory towns---consisting of over a hundred thousand souls---they were housed. Eight workers slept in one small dormitory room. Their jobs drove them to despair and death.

I pictured myself as one of those Chinese workers squinting on the assembly line. I held tweezers-size tools, inserting thousands of chips a day. Would I be able to survive just one eight-hour shift? I saw myself without friends or family with no relief from loneliness.

Monotony filled every minute of my long day on the factory line. Would I consider life worth living? Would I jump?

"In whose hands did these electronic devices end up?" I thought. "Do they care about me? My pain? My suffering? My existence?"

Like bats at dusk flying out of their guano-filled caves, I pictured a line of millions of paper airplanes—made up of American hundred-dollar bills—gliding across the Pacific and landing on the roof of my Beijing death factory.

That night I saw photographs on the *History Channel* of 10 year-old boys working long hours in West Virginia's coal mines or eleven year-old girls working in Lower Manhattan sweat shops sewing hundreds of garments a day. The coal was cheap as were the clothes manufactured in the US at the turn of the century. I felt good hearing that child labor laws have long been enforced in the States.

Then an advertisement for the movie, *Blood Diamonds* appeared on the screen. I recalled how African workers were treated as slaves in Sierra Leone's diamond mines, but I had not bought any of these conflict diamonds.

As I tried to rest my head on my pillow, I tossed and turned knowing the joy of holding, watching, listening to and playing with my brand new iPad 2 had vanished forever.

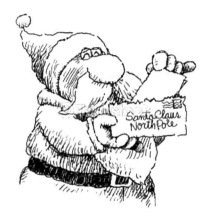

A Letter to Santa

By Keith Reaves

I can remember a time when I was visiting my parents, and out of an old dusty drawer my mother pulled a photo album. We were looking at old pictures and reminiscing about time gone by. An old letter I wrote to Santa when I was maybe six or seven years old fell from the back of the book. I looked at the letter and chuckled as I remarked, "Mom, my handwriting hasn't changed since I was seven."

I noticed that I was polite asking about Santa's family, how his wife and the reindeer were doing. I reminded him about how good I had been all year. Then I went for the kill and asked for a Hot Wheels track and race cars. It was like I was talking to an old friend or to a grandparent, or at least what I thought it would be, since I grew up without grandparents. After looking at the letter for awhile and thinking about the good memories, I carefully folded the letter and put it back in the dusty drawer and went on about my way.

Christmas has always been my favorite time of year to get together with family, celebrate the birth of Christ, eat lots of food, stand in long lines at the mall and receive and give gifts as well.

This got me thinking, now that I'm an adult, what would I say in a letter to Santa? If I had to give him a gift, what would it be? I would have to show my appreciation for all of the years Santa had been good to me. I usually received at least one thing I wanted even though I was sometimes not so nice. I couldn't give Santa something that I could purchase from the mall since Santa has access to every gift imaginable. I didn't want to give him something he would have no use for, so I would write him a letter and pass on some of the knowledge that I've learned over the years. The letter would go something like this:

Dear Santa,

Thank you for all of the gifts you provided me over the years even though, at times, I was more naughty than nice. I especially thank you for the 10-speed bike I received when I was 12 years old. I used it every day to ride back and forth to school, and it was a great source of exercise.

Santa, I also appreciate the fact that you are a senior citizen and still able to work. Climbing in and out of chimneys and carrying sacks full of toys is no easy task and the fact that you're still able to do it at your age is amazing! Please make sure when you're picking up the sacks of toys that you lift with your knees to save you from back strain.

Having a big belly that shakes like a bowl full of jelly when you laugh is also something that adds pressure to your back. It is also not healthy to carry fat in your midsection. It is a sign of obesity and could lead to high blood pressure and heart disease. Adding some cardio during the year and cutting fat from your diet should help trim down your stomach. One sign that you may be suffering from high blood pressure is those red rosy cheeks. Now those red cheeks could be from the cold, but it is a telltale sign of high blood pressure.

I know you have kids all over the world leaving you cookies and whole milk, but you don't have to eat at every stop. Try asking for vegetables like carrot sticks and celery, because vegetables metabolize better in the evening. A cookie once in a while is okay.

The one thing I love about you most, Santa, is your spirit of giving and your jolly attitude, but nowadays when you say ho, ho, ho to someone it takes on a different meaning. Take care of yourself Santa. We'll see you soon.

Love,

Keith

I think of those gifts of knowledge about lifting with your knees and not your back, watching what you eat and your weight, and watching for who you are calling a Ho is good advice and something that Santa will take into consideration. I hope it's not a letter he sticks into some dusty old drawer, but one that he'll find useful in his life from here on.

Keith Reaves is a native of New Jersey, having lived the last seven years in South Florida. He is presently a first year Barry University Graduate Student.

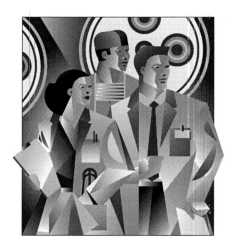

The Complete Diagnosis

By Clayton Jeans

I t's now been over a month since my second surgery and I can now walk upright – kind of.

Hot dog on a hamburger bun.

This is what it must have felt like to be Cro-Magnon man. But alas, life is close to normal. Except of course for the 10-inch cut I have up my stomach, which looks like a zipper because of the staples. Nevertheless, I'm out of the hospital and trying to return to normal life. Normal is a very loose term at this point. It is early March and the ride began in early January, so my "normal life" is more like a train wreck.

As mentioned before, I was first diagnosed with a tumor in the appendix. The medical term is a mixed adenocarinoma of the appendix, which had metastasized into the nearby lymph nodes. Out of 24 lymph nodes removed and tested with the hemicolectomy, only three came up positive with tumors. I was classified as Stage III Colon cancer because of the spread to the lymph nodes. It's hard to stomach that phrase at first when you hear it from a doctor.

"You have Stage III Colon Cancer, any questions??" Yeah – can you slap me to make sure I'm awake!

Keep in mind, this is stage III out of IV.

It's kinda nice starting closer to the top. Similar to being named Vice-President with no prior experience!

As mentioned before, I am lucky. All of this was discovered by the grace of God. I was fortunate enough to have a tumor create a blockage in my appendix, which eventually led to the appendicitis. We are talking about millimeters of space here. If this tumor was a few clicks left or right, it could have ended up real bad.

The primary tumor was in the process of moving out of my appendix. The pathology results showed the primary tumor piercing through the cell lining, on its way to God knows where, to do only God knows what.

Talk about an uninvited guest who drinks all your liquor, eats all your food and then kicks your dog...

I could have gone on for years as normal, all the while these tumors would be growing and spreading around my body, but I didn't. I got appendicitis instead. Appendicitis is cool.

Thanks tumor!

After all the surgeries were complete and I was able to walk again, Dr. Ratliff recommended I go speak with an oncologist. He recommended a friend at his hospital. He also recommended that I seek a second opinion no matter what his colleague concluded. My parents went ahead and got me in at another hospital to speak with another oncologist.

The goal for me now was to find out what the surgical results were and try to sew my life back together. But of course, the next few steps along the timeline were not as simple as that.

My single hope was that both oncologists would come to the same conclusions and recommend the same course of action. I didn't care what the conclusions would be as much as I simply wanted to know. At least if they both concluded bad news, I would have some control over what my next few moves would be. This is all I wanted.

However, since nothing in my life is straight forward, the recommendations were different. Typical – more confusion. The first oncologist told me the tumors that spread were very small and since they were located in the closest lymph nodes to my appendix, there is a minimal chance they had spread anywhere else. I was pronounced healthy and sent on my way.

OUTSTANDING! That guy is getting a Christmas card.

All I needed to do now is go hear the same news from another oncologist, so I could finally put all of this nonsense to bed.

Enter MD Anderson – the Mecca of Cancer research and treatment. I was scheduled to see Dr. Paulo Hoff, (or as I like to call him – the Hoffmeister), another oncologist to go over my pathology results. He told me the same things as the other doctor, confirming the results of the pathology examination.

RAD!

He confirmed the spread was only to three local lymph nodes and that the likelihood anything else was in my body was very low.

Of course doc, tell me something I don't already know.

Well, I shouldn't have been so cocky, because he did tell me something I didn't know – and it was something I wasn't happy to hear.

He was concerned with several things. Number one, he was concerned about my age. It seems I am quite young for this type of cancer, in this particular location of the body. The doctors wanted to be more aggressive than usual with their diagnosis and recommendation due to this fact.

He was also concerned about the way the primary tumor spread. As mentioned before, the primary tumor was located in the appendix. It contained three types of cancerous cells--carcinoid, adenocarcinoma, and signet ring cells. For those of you who are not oncologists let me just tell you--this combination is rare and damned perplexing to the doctors.

So it seems I am now the poster boy for "how the hell did this happen" in the medical field. I am still waiting for my Barbara Walters interview...

Out of the three, the signet ring cells and adenocarcinoma are the most aggressive and dangerous of the bunch. That is not to say the carcinoid can't kill you, it will simply just do it slower than the others.

What ended up happening in my case is that only the carcinoid cells spread to my lymph nodes. This apparently is highly unusual, since the most aggressive types (adenocarcinoma and signet ring cell) of neuroendocrine tumors were in the primary. The doctors have such little statistical information for such a strange case, they seem to be shooting from the hip with everything they tell me.

Nice to know I am so unique and special!

I actually have my picture on the wall of "Jacked Up" at the hospital. It is right next to the guy who won the Annual Cafeteria Taco Eating contest – not sure if I'm supposed to feel proud about that...

Anyway, the doctor was concerned as to why this least aggressive cancer cell spread to my lymph nodes alone. He wanted me to undergo a series of diagnostic tests to make sure there was nothing they missed in the surgeries. ☀

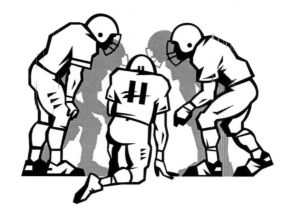

Breaking Into Medicine

By Austin L. Lyman

R ed Dawn arrived. And like a young Patrick Schwayze, I faced staggering odds. Before me stood a towering row of three large linebackers, each huffing and puffing like a Minotaur ready to knock my block off. Drops of sweat slipped off the black hair above the napes of their necks escaping from their helmets like limestone dripping off a stalagtite. During this brief hiatus, the sun at their back bore into my helmet, pushing beads of sweat over my eyes and onto my chapped lips. I watched my opponents engorge themselves with water and electrolytes as they desperately tried to cool down between each exercise.

Soon enough, they were prepared. I tracked the red-shirted ball carrier prancing behind his herd. And at the whistle blow, I sprang from my stance with a clenched jaw, raised head and outstretched fists. My hooves buried deep into the ground as I attempted to embrace the image of a barreling black bull bent towards his antagonist. But like a pinball, I bounced between the tactical, unabated hits from all sides and landed backwards on my tail in the wet grass.

Boos and cheers erupted from teammates as I gathered my legs underneath me. My fingers dug into the dirt beneath the grass as I balanced with my two feet like a tripod in order to lift myself up, but my quick recovery signaled the bullies to pounce once more.

SNAP! The earth failed to soften my fall. And suddenly, an unfamiliar, warm flare of pain surged throughout my wrist. My pulse carried the pain to my brain's protopathic centers. I winced, sending beads of sweat and tears running down my cheeks. Slowly rolling onto my knees, I cradled my left wrist as if holding an egg. I felt my body going into shock as I watched my hand's resting tremor mimic Tom Hank's character in the movie "Saving Private Ryan."

The bone had almost broken through my skin, which ballooned out. I knelt, stared and examined my arm's lameness. I feared the look on my parents faces about what I had done to myself. I feared the thought of social impotence—cut from the football team. I never considered the gravity of an injury. For me, the biggest risk about football was a bad headache or disappointing my overly fanatic football-fan of a father.

Then, my coach walked over and stood above me, "Get up son. Time to get back in the ring," he commanded lifting me by my shoulder pads. My mouth opened but, my eyes, pointing downward, spoke the words. Upon the sight of the puffy protrusion from my arm, he yelled, "Trainer!"

Amidst the hum of the cold A/C, I searched the white concrete walls of the athletic trainer's office, scanning the grotesque figures printed on posters. As an eighth grader, human anatomy had previously limited itself to the skin's shallow surface, so I felt fascinated by these detailed artistic displays. They resembled the road maps Dad kept in the car. Upon locating a skinned, red Adonis cartoon, I scooted off my blue bed one leg at a time for a closer look. Blue highways ran up and down the arm, weaving over and under osseous medians. I noticed the same cerulean lines running under my skin. I struggled to interpret the definitions of life printed in the black Roman text over the red muscles and white bones. The unfamiliar words mixed in my mind like a cerebral stew of terms: distal, proximal, flexor, extensor. I had no idea what they meant, but it sure looked important.

Moments later, footsteps clicked outside the door, and I scurried back to the bed. Seated with my legs dangling and arm cradled against my chest, the door cracked open. A voice superseded a patriotic wardrobe of long white socks, mid-thigh, blue chino shorts and a short-sleeve red polo featuring our school's bucking *bos taurus*.

"Honey, I'm afraid you're gonna need to get some x-rays," bellowed our trainer, Ms. Smith. Her strong, syrupy southern drawl fortified her already intimidating 5-foot-11-inch stocky build and pixy brown hairstyle. She parked my wrist between two aluminum bars and silky sleeve wrap. Then, I watched Ms. Smith wrap athletic tape around another player's ankle. Her figure-eight fashion flew furiously fast and without hesitation. She flung her two hands in focused, coordinated 5-step movements.

Soon, I fell into my new routine: I reported every other weekday morning before school to Ms. Smith's office where I joined teammates, some of whom were also rehabbing their joints. I began my rehab exercises. With each tug and turn, my wrist screamed, "What are you doing that for?" But my wrist wasn't the only one with questions.

Intrigued by another student's hopping on one foot, I asked, "What's the benefit for that exercise, Ms. Smith?"

"He's working on strengthening his *peroneus longus* muscles," she replied.

"Peronist?" I asked, "Isn't that some political party in Argentina?"

Ultimately, my visits conjured more and more questions, bringing Ms. Smith to a boil, "Listen, hon. How about you come back here after school during practice, and I'll teach ya about training while you help me with these water coolers and my gear?"

I accepted her bid to barter. And like a calf to a steer, I followed Ms. Smith into the realm of athletic training.

Later that evening, as I stood in front of the school building, I rubbed my hand over the tips of my opposing fingers to stay warm. In the humid, cold air, I looked around to see the same three, large linebackers aligned in their row. This time none stood huffing or puffing, but rather, sat beside their steaming helmets benign and battered from the day's long training, carefully holding out their elbows and knees like chicken wings. Ms. Smith posted herself before them like a towering Theseus. From a distance, I felt an excitement over their oncoming discomfort from the alcohol pads that would come in contact with their fresh wounds.

"Revenge!" I thought. Then, I witnessed the three bullies reach out for an appreciative clap, one firm hand shake and words of thanks for Ms. Smith as they ran back onto the field. Glancing at the white padded squares taped on their skin, my hand ran back and forth over my cast. I felt Stallone's message wrapped over my wrist: in the realm of sports medicine, "It isn't about how hard you hit, it is about how hard you can get hit and keep moving forward." It's about how many cuts, scrapes and breaks you take and keep pursuing your mission. I grabbed the heavy bags weighed down by spools of Coban, prewrap and ice bags and walked back toward the field, toward my team, toward my patients.

Austin L. Lyman is a bio-med graduate student at Barry University.

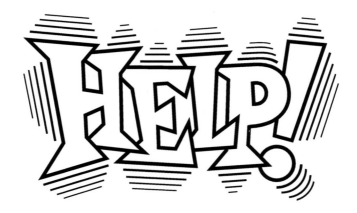

I exited the grocery store and saw an old lady with no legs seated in a wheelchair just beyond the doorway. She stopped me as I walked out, and she asked me to give her a ride across town. She was dirty and old with unkempt salt and pepper hair. Her face was gaunt. Her parched, dark orange-peel skin barely covered the bones beneath it. Several teeth were missing. I smelled the alcohol and tobacco from six feet away.

"Please, I just need to go to Martin Luther King Boulevard. You could drop me at Marvin's Rib Shack."

"I'm very sorry," I replied to this stranger. "I'm in a hurry. If I had time, I'd be happy to take you there. Here, take this dollar for bus fare." I walked off, wishing I could have done more.

About two weeks later, this same old woman was sitting in her wheelchair in the building where I worked, the district office of the Florida Department of Health and Rehabilitative Services. She may have been inquiring about some sort of public assistance. She was sweaty, her usual disheveled self, and she was looking for a ride.

"Hey, I remember you. Can you carry me over to Martin Luther King Boulevard? I'd really appreciate it." She smacked her lips. I imagined she spent a lot of time trying to convince people to drive her somewhere. There was a young girl with her, perhaps twenty-five years old, pushing her wheelchair.

"How'd you get here?" I asked.

The young girl said, "We rode the wheelchair bus." She was hard of hearing and had a bit of a lisp, so "bus" sounded like "bush."

The secretary in our office witnessed the exchange, and I asked if she knew this legless woman in the wheelchair, who seemed to have a knack for getting around town. Bobbie said, "Yeah, she hangs around the bars in Frenchtown. Her name is Flora Mae. She's always bumming money and rides from people."

Regardless of how I might have felt about her lifestyle--she still reeked of cheap booze and cigarettes--I felt bad about not giving her a ride before. I had time now.

Flora reminded me of a time years ago when I was in college. There was an old man with no legs who was mobile only because he had one of those hardwood platforms with wheels under him. He always played harmonica just outside the place where I did my banking. With gloved hands and a smile on his face, he seemed to be able to push himself anywhere he needed to be. Other than his smile, like Flora, he had a weathered old face with scraggly salt and pepper hair. I had many opportunities to watch him in action and make a contribution in exchange for his musical services. He placed a rusting coffee tin-can in front of him for donations.

One Friday, I walked into the bank to cash my paycheck and make a deposit. The old, legless man had wheeled himself into the bank and was in line to make a deposit of his "donations." He had two large-sized coffee cans full of coins and dollar bills sitting next to him on his wheeled platform.

My first thought was, "Wow, he earns a lot of cash playing his harmonica." He used what skills and talents he had to earn his way in the world, and I didn't mind contributing to his cause when I was able.

Flora Mae had her own set of skills and talents that she used to convince others to help her. Flora had a gift to play on people's sympathies.

I helped Flora and the young girl into my car. I folded her wheelchair and stowed it in the trunk. The young, partially deaf, girl thanked me. As I drove them to MLK Boulevard, it occurred to me, I knew Flora. She had been part of a syphilis investigation I had done a year or two prior to this. She was also a crack addict.

Flora, never at a loss for conversation, explained she lost her legs due to diabetes. "I got all sorts of diseases and afflictions. Yeah, I practically live at the hospital...there and the health department."

I dropped them off and asked the girl, "Do you need a ride anywhere?"
She said, "No, I'll hang out there and push Flora around for awhile."
"Do you live around here?"

"No." She replied, so I gave her bus fare and drove away.

Dropping Flora and the young girl off wasn't the end of this story. About a month later, I read the obituaries: *Flora Mae Cromarte, 41, of 657 Washington Street, died Friday at Tallahassee Memorial Hospital of heart failure.*

The obit stunned me. I always thought Flora was at least sixty or sixty-five years old. Life hit her pretty hard. There was a separate article in the paper with a picture of Flora's life-warn face, a broad smile and missing front teeth. She was staring right into the camera. Apparently, a lot of Tallahasseans knew Flora Mae. According to the write-up, she was homeless, stubborn, diabetic, handicapped and had heart problems. The reporter omitted her alcoholism and drug addiction.

Regardless of her lifestyle, I was happy to be one of the strangers to have given her a ride, just as I was glad to help the harmonica man. I realized that we all have special skills and talents for earning our way in the world. And then I thought about Blanche DuBois in *Streetcar Named Desire*, that the two of them could always depend on the kindness of strangers.

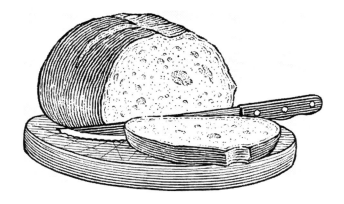

A Close Call

By Mort Laitner

A t 5:00 pm, Lefty, Joel, Allen and I ran home while waving and yelling, "Good-bye," to the Camp Alamac staff and counselors. My friends and I headed toward the village with our stomachs still full from lunch and our heads still full of ideas on how we would spend the final four hours of our day.

We strolled down the Glen Wild Road pretending to be pirates ready to launch a murderous raid on the town. We swung invisible swords and dueled with each other. Joel ringed his fingers into the shape of a spyglass scanning Kreiger's Garage and Gas Station as if looking for victims to plunder, while Lefty pulled back the string from his imaginary bow and shot arrows at the sun. Then Allen, my redhead friend, with a Froggy voice and a freckled face, started to sing:

"Ninety-nine bottles of beer on the wall,
Ninety-nine bottles of beer. Take one down and pass it around,
Ninety-eight bottles of beer on the wall."

The rest of us joined in and after three more bottles were passed around, I broke in with a barrage of questions, "What brand of beer was on that wall? Budweiser? Schlitz? What would happen if all those bottles fell off the wall? Who would clean up the mess?"

The threesome pondered their replies as if they were taking the New York State Regents Exam.

Breaking the silence, Lefty, our skinny historian, piped in, "Those bottles were on a pirate ship. In the old days bottles didn't have paper labels affixed to them. Therefore they had no brand."

"Yeah, Lefty's right. This is an old pirate song and the lowest mate on the ship would swab the room clean if any bottles hit the deck," Joel replied.

Allen, displaying his knowledge of pirate lingo, followed, "You'd have a bunch of mutinous pirates on your hands if all 99 bottles broke. Those buccaneers loved to drink their grog."

Turning onto Broadway, Joel switched tunes and bellowed,

"Row, row, row, your boat gently down the stream
Merrily, merrily, merrily, life is but a dream."

The rest of us, in our deepest voices, joined in with our arms flaying as if we were drunken sailors rowing the boat toward a pirate ship.

As eleven-year-olds, living in the Catskills, our lives were one big camp song. We sang loudly, as if no one lived in the village. We sang the tunes in the carefree voice of children without responsibilities. Our lives were all fun and games. What did we have to worry about? What harm could befall us?

I invited Joel, my best friend since kindergarten, to stop at my house for a Coke and as we stepped in the door, we yelled at our friends, "See you later alligator."

Lefty and Allen laughed and retorted, "In a while crocodile."

We entered my kitchen and saw my short, slightly over-weight grandmother, Babcia Roza, rendering chicken fat into schmaltz—the Yiddish word for fat. Like young sea hawks we watched as Grandma Rose held a sharp, bone-handled kitchen knife and trimmed the skin off the fat. She placed an eight-inch-high pile of uncooked chicken fat on a clear-plastic chopping block. We watched as she chopped the fat into small pieces. Then she dropped the pieces into a large black frying pan and added slices of onions. As she cooked the concoction over low heat, the smell of oil permeated our nostrils. Magically the fat turned to oil. Grandma stirred the mixture as the fat began to brown.

When the white fat disappeared, she used her slotted wooden spoon to remove the crispy chicken fat skin bits—gribenes—a tasty treat for which we anxiously waited. The schmaltz remained in the frying pan until Grandma poured it into a glass-mason jar and placed it in the refrigerator. In a few hours it would be ready to spread on bread.

After guzzling our Cokes, Joel and I decided to take archery practice in Lefty's backyard. In my room, I found my nylon bow and leather quiver filled with six hunting arrows. Each hunting arrow had a razor-sharp, three-inch steel blade. These arrows were designed to kill deer.

Lefty's backyard consisted of a small field where we played touch football; a wooded area where we dug for worms, had crab apple and snow ball fights; and a narrow path that led to Lefty's Dad's shoe store.

From one end of the field, Joel and I took turns shooting our steel-tipped arrows into a fifty-year-old maple tree. Impressed with our dead-eye accuracy, we crossed the field to remove the deeply-embedded, razor-sharp arrows from the bark.

Having tired of shooting at tree trunks, we decided to have a contest to see who could shoot their hunting arrow the highest. Joel shot first. He pulled back the string, tightly securing the arrow between his thumb and index finger and arching his bow with all the muscle an eleven-year-old could muster. Joel let go and his arrow zoomed seventy-five feet straight up in the air. Within three seconds, the arrow flipped over and jettisoned toward the ground before landing point first, within ten feet from where we stood. We gasped, inhaling lungs full of air, realizing the extreme danger of this fool-hardy game.

A taste of fear filled my mouth, my esophagus, my whole digestive track, but I would not be dissuaded from taking my shot.

It was my turn. I wanted to shoot my arrow higher than Joel's. I flexed my bow, placed the pronged plastic arrow tip between its nylon string, and pulled back with all my might, releasing my pinched fingers and letting the arrow soar.

As soon as I let it go, I glanced down field and saw Lefty's Dad slowly walking toward us. I heard Joel gasp. My lips froze, as my eyes prayed that the razor-sharp hunting arrow would not puncture Lefty's Dad's skull. I watched in horror as the arrow flipped and headed toward earth.

In those three seconds I knew my "fun-and-game life" would end in tragedy. Then the arrow landed point first in the ground—ten feet behind Lefty's Dad. I exhaled, as I heard Joel whisper, "Holy cow, that was close! We're not playing this game any more."

In silence, I watched Lefty's father walk toward and enter his house. He never would know how close he came to death. I stepped foreword, walked across the field and pulled the arrow out of the ground. I examined the arrow. I examined my life—as well as any eleven-year-old could—and reaffirmed my belief in the Almighty.

Leaving the backyard with my bow and quivering knees, I whimpered, "Joel, I'm going home. I'll see you later."

At 9:00 pm, Joel stopped by my house to see how I was doing. He greeted my mom, who responded by opening her purse and giving us thirty-five cents to purchase fresh, right-out-of-the-oven-seeded-rye bread from Mortman's Bakery. She knew how much we loved the warm bread.

As we ran to the bakery, Joel and I smelled the freshly-baked breads from a block away. We ordered, paid, and watched as the noisy old bread slicer cut though the loaf. Mrs. Mortman placed the rye in a waxed-paper bag. Leaving the bakery, we politely said, "Thanks," as I clung to our treasure.

Exiting Mortman's, I ripped open the bag grabbing the tip of the loaf. We strolled back to the house sharing and devouring slice after slice. I watched half the loaf disappear.

We sang no camp songs, as our mouths were filled with rye.

Entering the kitchen, I remembered the schmaltz and quickly removed it from the refrigerator. With a bone-handled knife, I spread the schmaltz evenly across the face of two slices of bread, and I handed one to Joel. Biting into the slice of bread, I silently counted my blessings.

I would never tell this story to anyone because I didn't want to be labeled an idiot or face the wrath of Lefty's father. Instead, I preferred to remember the delicious taste of my grandmother's schmaltz spread across warm rye bread. ✵

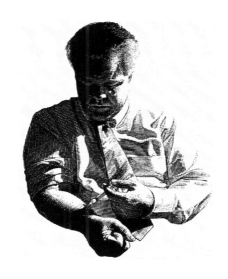

Meant to Be

By Randa Obid

Reflecting upon myself,
I do not like the person staring back at me.

I'm looking for absolution, living in a world of mass confusion.

These Age lines define
The scars of my past but I still deny
That this has become my life.

I've come to learn that "fate" is just an invention
With the intention to cover up the feeling of living an empty life.

I remember when I was a rose amongst the weeds,
I arose with a purpose to be the best that I can be.

That was the life I was meant to lead,
But then somehow I stumbled upon Methamphetamine.

I was once a rose who arose, I had risen, and then suddenly...

I started falling…

Falling fast, falling hard…

I fell short of my potential.
I had become infatuated with the crystal.

It started with an ingestion
Then an injection
Then an addiction.

What felt like days suddenly turned into years
My life slipped away. I couldn't even recognize myself in the mirror.
I was too distracted by the sensation of the cascading release
of dopamine,
To see that I lost everything.

So you see,
I have seen the way "fate" has teased me.
Does fate really want me to think, "it was all meant to be" as if
mentally
I should accept that this atrocity was meant for me
Because what's meant to be is to be empty?

Defined by the mistakes of my past:
I can never escape
From this jail I am in figuratively
Also literally.
Trapped here after what became of me-
A junkie who did desperate things for money
And now I am behind bars with nothing but me, myself
and my memories.

*Randa Obid is a Bio Med graduate student at Barry University working on a
Master's degree.*

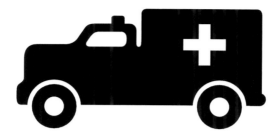

Twenty-Six Minutes

By Angie Hargot

Past the walls of volumes
analyzing atheism, polytheism. Existentialism. The Bible as metaphors.
Tomes of things that happened
and things that likely didn't.
Two decades spent searching for answers.
My hands trembled through the little white jewelry box.
My finger wrapped in the little band, I grasped it to keep it from
slipping, holding onto it
As if God,
or the authorities,
or Satan himself
for that matter
were to appear before me,
my soul the only means to save his life,
millimeters of metal would prove my willingness to sacrifice it.
If God exists
(but just never answers)
I would pry open his front door with spotless will.

It was in the inky recesses of Sunday. Six a.m.
The room so silent the ears began to ring a bit
the world so still, every passer-by bird
shocked.

His long howl shattered
the thickly-curtained bedroom
I scrambled for the tiny light switch
The dim glow revealed him
His muscles utterly tensed
His limbs contorted uncontrollably
violently shaking.
A bloody foam poured through his clenched jaw.

His eyes were transfixed at an angle, as if towards the past,
Blue as the walls of ancient Egyptian tombs,
the cold color of dreams
in them, a look of tortured sadness.
Of a mind battling, battling, against a stolen control.
I met them, but wasn't seen.

I asked over and over again if he was OK, my voice rising, as if it
would make him hear.

His arm gestured rapidly, inexplicably
Uncontrollably.
As if to asking for pen and paper to write
or as if to say
'CHECK PLEASE'
to the waiter across a congested restaurant.
But behind his eyes
he was filled with fear.

For minutes,
moments,
hours,
minutes.

My shaking fingers scarcely dialed the numbers

His mind a magnet struck by a hammer
not ready to pay the bill,

he struggled.
Unsuccessfully.

He gurgled. Spasmed.
and slipped away from me.

As still as an anniversary butterfly, he stopped breathing.

I moaned, and shook him violently. I swept the crimson foam from
his mouth.

The voice on the phone was calm with the sickening experience.
I fought it, too, my voice harsh and cold
with the cruelty that only a shredded heart can muster.
"Where ARE they?" I begged. "It's been so long."

I hug up the phone.

He choked and exhaled.
A fine spray of blood painted my face,
a sick Grail,
like the purple ink of the Byzantium.
The air filled his lungs again, but his eyes stayed shuttered.

Twenty-six minutes later, uniforms filled the room. He regained
consciousness,
surrounded by strangers.
He knew his name. Where he was.

"Do you know who this is?" They asked him.
"Of course I do — That's my wife." He said.
"What's her name?" They asked him.

He did not have an answer.

*Angie Hargot has a Bachelors degree in journalism from Florida International
University.*

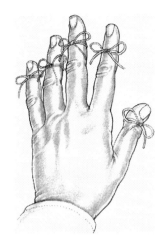

After The Stroke

By Deborah DeNicola

Often she speaks of a mysterious They. "When are They coming?"
"Where are they?" "Do they all do that, wear that, eat that?
"Must we pay Them?" But she forgets everything in a matter of minutes:
rooms, news, rules of a favorite card game. And she forgets she forgets.

Objects, once familiar, disappear, surface again in surprising places:
scotch tape in the medicine cabinet, jewelry under the sink, cash
in the refrigerator drawer. Still she wants to help me in the kitchen.
Sets the table with folded wax paper and sheets of foil for napkins.

I can fool her, tell her apple juice with ice is scotch on the rocks.
But she sneaks chocolate pudding for breakfast. On TV, watches
cartoons or the Spanish soaps. Her hair, which she always wore
in a neat French knot, is loose and sparse down her shoulders.
Her eyes grow small and dim in a thinning face, although,

some vanity remains intact. She applies mascara to her eyebrows,
powders wrinkles flat, blushes her nose, loops a scarf in a buttonhole,
clutches an evening bag to her bath robe. Her daughters
have her sisters' names. Old friends no longer call.

Each night she strings different words in a chain and repeats them
150 times. Sometimes there's a question she means to ask
but she can't find a sentence. Sparks and sputters instead.
She wants to go home when she is home. And when angry
with me, my mother hisses I hope you live this long. ☼

First published in Anderbo Online 2007

*Deborah DeNicola's most recent publications are The Future That Brought Her
Here; Memoir of a Call to Awaken, Nicholas Hays Press 2009, and her sixth book
of poetry Original Human, Word Tech Communications, 2010. Deborah edited
Orpheus & Company; Contemporary Poems on Greek Mythology, and, among other
award, received an NEA Fellowship*

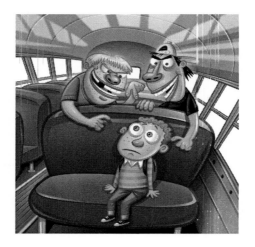

The Bully

By Liz Brady

There is a little voice inside
A bully
Relentless
Merciless
Cruel

Instead of fighting back
You take it
Believe it
Agree

It is time
For a revolution

When you no longer cower
The berating will stop

You can tell the bully
To go back to hell
You don't live there anymore

You can give him
Compassion no one ever showed
Heal him with kindness

You can stop reacting
Ignore him until he learns
He's wasting his time

But you can't keep encouraging him
Or pretending
You don't hear him

Harassment will follow you
It will get worse
Will cause destruction
Someone or something will break

Choose a path to healing
Make a plan
Be brave

All public institutions
Implemented anti-bullying policies
Make one
Follow it
Reclaim your power

You deserve the right to be happy
You deserve the right to be at peace
To piece together
What you've done right
Where you've gone wrong
Who you have hurt
How you can do better

Forgive yourself
Forgive the bully

And for your own sake
Stop beating yourself up

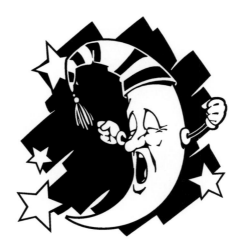

Insomnia

By Connie Goodman-Milone

Awake upon this
ceaseless night,
as stars burn on
through the twilight.
I sleep not now
as I once did then,
will my soul ever
find slumber again?

Connie Goodman-Milone, MSW is a Miami writer, hospice volunteer and co-author of bereavement poetry anthology. This poem appeared in <u>Walk A Giant Piano</u> (chapbook)

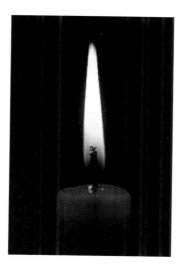

Candle in My Dark

By Rita Fidler Dorn

You were the candle in my dark.
You were the picnic in my park.
You were the music of my soul.

You helped me learn to make my way;
You taught me to structure every day.
You were the one who made me whole.

We cooked, we laughed, we went on cruises;
You gave me praise and kissed my bruises.
You told me I must always have a goal.

Your humor and your raunchy jokes
Laughter from our hearts evoked.
You played piano: classics, jazz, and rock 'n roll.

You loved my poems but hated my sewing;
Your all-time motto was, "Gotta keep going!"
You ate pickled herring on an onion roll.

Confidant, role model, opinion giver;
Brisk and sweet as a cool, spring river.
In my dreams, you will never grow old.

You were the candle in my dark.
You were the picnic in my park.
My memories of you will never grow cold.

Written in memory of my mother,
Beatrice Greenberg Fidler 1911-2000.

Ricki Dorn, an adjunct professor at Miami-Dade College and at Florida
International University, has been writing poetry since she was seven years old.
She presented a lecture workshop at the 2011 Mango Writers Conference in Miami,
entitled "How to Kickstart Your Own Creativity" and currently has two poetry
books in the works.

History of
Public Health
In Florida

FOREWORD

From the Senior Vice President of the Florida Medical Association

When H. Frank Farmer, Jr., M.D., Ph.D., was appointed in 2011 by Governor Rick Scott as State Surgeon General and State Health Officer in charge of the Florida Department of Health, he became the 25th State Health Officer in Florida's history.

The term "State Health Officer" first appeared in Florida law with the creation of the State Board of Health by the Florida Legislature in 1889. The Florida Constitution of 1885 had called for the establishment of the State Board of Health. The inclusion of this provision in the state constitution was led by a delegate to the constitutional convention, a President of the Florida Medical Association, John P. Wall, M.D., who is known as the Father of the State Board of Health. Dr. Wall's wife and young son had tragically succumbed to yellow fever in Tampa in 1871. So he became the prime mover to create a State Board of Health. The Legislature enacted it when Governor Francis Fleming called the Legislature into special session in February of 1889 in response to the yellow fever epidemic the year before in Jacksonville. The State Health Officer, who was required in the new law to be a doctor of medicine and a graduate of a recognized medical school, was invested by the Legislature with the power to enforce the public health laws of Florida.

This position of paramount importance to the state was first held by Joseph Yates Porter, M.D., who was the second longest serving State Health Officer, 28 years from 1889 to 1917. Dr. Porter, who had been President of the Florida Medical Association in 1886, developed the State Board of Health on the strong foundation of his outstanding leadership and vision. He constructed the first permanent headquarters building for the State Board of Health in Jacksonville on land donated by the city to house Florida's first health department.

The longest serving State Health Officer was Wilson T. Sowder,

M.D., M.P.H. who served 29 years from 1945 to 1974. Dr. Sowder expanded Florida's county health departments to all 67 counties during his long tenure, in which he retained his commission in the United States Public Health Service. He is well deserving of the many accolades bestowed on him by public health authorities for forging Florida's statewide public health system, at both state and county levels, into one of the finest in the nation. Dr. Sowder wrote a comprehensive history of his service in public health in Florida spanning the terms of eleven Governors.

The collection of contributions that appear in this publication are by the State Health Officers who came after Dr. Sowder, starting with E. Charlton Prather, M.D., M.P.H. in 1974. They tell the story of how the State Board of Health was abolished in 1969 without the previous constitutional provision protecting it, as that provision had been eliminated the preceding year; how the state headquarters was moved to Tallahassee after becoming part of the huge social services agency, the Department of Health and Rehabilitative Services (HRS); and how after a quarter of a century of efforts, led by Florida Senator William G. "Doc" Myers, M.D. of Hobe Sound, and with the strongest support and advocacy of the Florida Medical Association, the Florida Public Health Association, and others, public health was reborn with the unanimous creation of the new Department of Health by the Florida Legislature in 1996.

This was an epic advancement for public health to address 21st century challenges. Alvin E. Smith, M.D., President of the Florida Medical Association at that time, worked closely with the leadership in the Florida House of Representatives and Florida Senate to enact the Senator William G. "Doc" Myers Public Health Act of 1996. Former State Health Officer, James T. Howell, M.D., M.P.H., and other public health leaders worked tirelessly to establish a singular Department of Health, similar to the State Board of Health that had served Florida so well from 1889 to 1969. Dr. Howell was then appointed as the first Secretary of the new Department of Health and State Health Officer by Governor Lawton Chiles. The title of State Health Officer was thus restored to its present status as head of the state's public health department.

It has been my honor to have worked directly for Dr. Charlton

Prather as the Legislative Liaison for the Division of Health beginning in 1974, and then with his successor, Dr. James Howell, during the first of his three terms as State Health Officer commencing in 1979. Later, in my capacity on the staff of the Florida Medical Association starting in 1984, I have known and been associated with all of Dr. Prather's and Dr. Howell's successors, especially Charles S. Mahan, M.D., Robert G. Brooks, M.D., M.P.H., John Agwunobi , M.D., M.P.H., Ana Viamonte Ros, M.D., M.P.H., and with present State Surgeon General and State Health Officer, H. Frank Farmer, Jr., M.D., Ph.D., who served as President of the Florida Medical Association in 2001-02.

Our State Health Officers have protected and improved the public health of our citizens and visitors through their knowledge and leadership as physicians for our statewide community. They are particularly responsible for making Florida a healthier place to live and visit, as it has grown exponentially to become the nation's fourth most populous state. Dr. Porter and Dr. Sowder would be very proud that their legacies in Florida have been continued so ably by all of the outstanding physicians who have held the vitally important position of State Health Officer.

E. Russell Jackson, Jr.

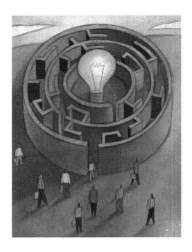

A Marvelous Career*

E. Charlton Prather, M.D., M.S., M.P.H.
State Health Officer
July 1974 – July 1979 and May 1985 – December 1986

The early years were among the most tumultuous of the State public health organization's 90 year history. The 1969 revision of the State Constitution (the first since 1886) abolished the State Board of Health (established in 1889) and stripped the State Health Officer of all authority.

The State Board of Health (SBH), the title both for the administrative and operational offices of the agency and the policy/rule making supervisory Board, became administrative services in the Department of Health and Rehabilitative Services (HRS). Some twenty-eight agencies and boards, all the human services of state government, were consolidated into twelve divisions of the new department. The policy-making board of the State Board of Health was abolished and became an advisory body to the new Secretary. Even earlier, the 1965 legislature transferred the state's mental health division out State Board of Health. Other losses at the time included the responsibility for narcotic control transferred to the Florida Bureau of Law Enforcement, the responsibility for air and water pollution to a new Department of Environmental Regulation, and dairy inspections and quality assurance of milk products to the Department of Agriculture. The advent of the federal Medicare and Medicaid programs removed the State Board of Health from most activities that gave medical care services to the indigent.

Even more drastic changes were wrought by the 1975 legislature reorganization of HRS. The Division of Health and its predecessor housed in Jacksonville since inception (1889) was ordered to relocate headquarters to Tallahassee. Divisions were abolished and became "Program Offices" under an Assistant Secretary for Planning. Operational responsibility of the original divisions were transferred to an Assistant Secretary for Operations. The statutory title of "State Health Officer" was abolished and authority transferred to the Secretary of the Department. (However, the Secretary under his authority, re-instated "State Health Officer" as a functional title to the Director of Health Program Office.) The law provided a third Assistant Secretary for Administration. Program offices were responsible only for planning programs, monitoring and quality assurance. The fundamental business activity of carrying out the planned programs became the responsibility of the Assistant Secretary of Operations. "Operations" were accomplished through 11 Districts; each with a "District Administrator" who was accountable to the Assistant Secretary of Operations.

Each "Program Office" was represented in the District by a "District Program Office" accountable to "District Administrator". County Health Departments, always the "delivery arm" of the State Public Health function, became the responsibility of the District Administrator. The District Health Program was headed by a "District Health Program Supervisor". There was no direct communication between the State Program Office and the local health departments.

The relocation of headquarter offices and reshuffling of staff resulted in many staff resignations. From some seven-hundred staff in Jacksonville, the greatly reorganized and redefined "Health Program Office" in Tallahassee began operation with a staff of fifty-eight. Many employees obtained employment within other activities of the Department in the Jacksonville area and elsewhere about the state, including Tallahassee. Many resigned and/or retired from state service.

The great majority of the fifty-eight staff had advanced degrees in one or more of the "public health sciences" – all "public health professionals" committed to the matters of health but none had training or experience in the "science of planning". Yet, a first priority was to develop integrated plans in which resources and expertise of the many previously separated agencies could be brought to bear in an integrated way upon any problem. NASA planners with Ph.D.s were brought in to guide us. The focus and object of the departmental efforts became the "client", not the "patient."

We had trouble reconciling septic tanks or epidemics as "clients". Such was entirely new to the public health terms. The "patient" for public health programming had always been the community. New ways of thinking were required. The demands were frustrating, yet "shoulders were put to the wheel" and all did the best they could. Emotional and physical stress was tremendous. Unsuccessful efforts to accomplish integrated programming as envisioned by statute caused the beginning of the dissolution and ultimate demise of HRS.

It was within this milieu that I became Director of the State Division of Health and State Health Officer on July 1, 1974. My predecessor, Wilson T. Sowder, M.D., M.P.H., Florida's longest serving State Health Officer, had developed over his twenty-eight plus years in office, a model state/local public health program recognized nationally and internationally. He had served as an expert consultant to the World Health Organization, the Pan American Health Organization, the U.S. Public Health Service and many states on matters of public health organization and programming. Even before I was appointed to the position of State Health Officer and serving as State Epidemiologist and Chief of the Bureau of Prevention Diseases, I hosted official visits from India's Secretary of Health for orientation into our systems of disease control and surveillance. I also hosted Victor Heiser, M.D., author of "American Doctor's Odyssey" who was referred here by the World Leprosy Foundation for "seeing" our leprosy surveillance system. Florida's local health service system was praised widely. There was a functioning local health department in each of the state's sixty-seven counties – all operating as cooperative efforts between state and county governments and mutually funded.

But all was changed by the reorganization act of 1976. Many long standing programs and essential support services were eliminated: Nursing, Nutrition, Health, Education, Research, Veterinary Public

Health, publication of an Annual Report, the "Florida Health Notes" (initiated in 1889), the public health library (the largest in the U.S.), a film collection of 100's of films, among other programs all disappeared.

It had been a proud organization with prideful employees. I was highly complimented to be chosen to head this outstanding, well running internationally recognized public health organization. (I never viewed myself a "replacement" for Dr. Sowder.) I consider myself the prime witness to the death of organized public health in Florida.

Yet some good things happened:

Widespread confusion about "how does public health fit" and "what really is its function" (Should it not be mainly the provision of medical/illness care services to the indigent, medical needy of Florida?) was widely discussed in this new coordinated and comprehensive way of offering human services in Florida.

The Secretary directed that a special study be undertaken. A panel of distinguished public health experts and sociologists from around the nation, along with administrators, physicians and citizens was gathered. Sequestered in an out-of-town location, the group considered most every facet of public health programming, administration, and funding within the present organizational environment. Many good recommendations resulted. A particular one addressed establishment of a uniform public health program with stated performance standards, defined target populations and measurable outcomes. Health Program Office staff immediately set to work in collaboration with staff from District Offices and County Health Units (CHU) to develop, test, implement and refine an automated management system that satisfied legislative intent as well as meet all HRS goals and objectives.

It was two years after I left (the first time) that the "CHU Management System" became fully operational and provided timely information for a wide variety of state, local and national applications. James T. Howell, MD., M.P.H. was then Director of the Health Program Office.

In spite of those tedious, stressful and often frustrating times of the early years of the 1976 HRS re-configuration, many improvements in public health programs offering occurred.

- The '76 legislature provided for Diabetes Treatment and Research Centers at the three medical schools.

- A radiation control program was established and radiological technologists certified.
- The Phenylketonuria legislation was amended to include additional genetic and metabolic diseases.
- The Federal Safe Drinking Water Act directed that water supplies be tested for toxic chemicals and radionuclides.
- The Family Planning Program was greatly expanded with new federal funds.
- The Women, Infant and Children (WIC) Program was expanded to all CHU's and Improved Pregnancy Outcome projects initiated is selected areas.

My job in most of these was simply signing the papers presented by staff.

Nothing impressive or particularly memorable comes to mind from my second tenure as Director of the Health Program and State Health Officer. My job was mostly "house keeping" after Dr. Howell left following his second term in the position. I formally retired following 35 years, 6 months, 27 days and 1.5 hours with the Florida State Public Health organization. And a marvelous career it was!!

Postscript:

Even before 1986, HRS was beginning to fall apart. Several of the pre-1976 independent agencies that were incorporated into the new mammoth department had already been split off as new departments or programs in other existing organizations. Notably were Corrections, Vocational Rehabilitation, Blind Services, and others. By 1997 only three of the original 28 agencies remained: Social Services, Mental Health and Public Health. That year, largely thorough the efforts of the Florida Medical Association, Public Health was split out and became the Florida Department of Health. Mental Health and Social Services were renamed the Department of Children and Families – The HRS was no more.

* It has been some 25 years since I retired. Memory is fuzzy. A lot of these memories reported here have been brought to mind by Dr. William Bigler's paper

Public Health in Florida – Yesteryear Florida's Public Health Centennial

Published in the Florida Journal of Public Health, Vol. 1, No. 3, May, 1989, p. 7-19

With Dr. Bigler's permission his words have been used liberally.

The reader is referred there for a marvelous recounting of Florida's public health story. ✵

E. Charlton Prather, M.D., M.P.H., M.S.
A note or two about me

I'm a Floridian by birth; born and grew up in Jasper, Hamilton County, Florida. Attended the University of Florida. Graduated with Degree in Microbiology. Graduated work (in microbiology) was accomplished through a cooperative program between the University and the Laboratories of the Florida State Board of Health in Jacksonville in which class room study was accomplished on campus and "hands-on" work and research in the Jacksonville laboratories. Paul De Kruif's book "Microbe Hunters" convinced me while I was in the ninth grade that I was going to pursue a career in public health hunting microbes! The work in the state labs clinched the decision!

A Ph.D. in Microbiology (that's what Dr. De Kruif had!) was planned. But my mentor, Director of the Laboratories, Albert V. Hardy, M.D., Dr. P.H., a renowned Epidemiologist, convinced me otherwise – I attended Medical School at Wake Forest University.

I returned to the Florida State Board of Health, served an Internship in Public Health at the Jackson Memorial Hospital, and three years residency training in public health with the Board of Health.

I attended the School of Public Health, University of North Carolina, and graduated with a M.P.H. in Epidemiology. While there, I took advanced courses in Biostatistics. I was privileged to attend the CDC's four-week Epidemic Intelligence Service ("EIS") course in Atlanta.

The Board of Health saw fit to appoint me to the position of State Epidemiologist while I was attending the School of Public Health. After some seven years in the position, the Board elevated me to the position of Chief of the Bureau of Preventable Diseases. There, my responsibilities included the venereal diseases, immunization programming, zoonoses control, radiological health, occupational health, tuberculosis control, and epidemiology.

I continued to serve as the State Epidemiologist. Then in 1974, upon retirement of the state's longest serving State Health Officer, Dr. Wilson T. Sowder, I was chosen by the Secretary of the Department of Health and Rehabilitative Services and Governor Askew to head up the Division of Health; two years later to become the "Health Program Office".

Then at the end of 1986, I retired.

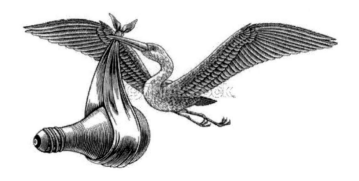

The Rebirth
of the Department
# of Health

James T. Howell, M.D., M.P.H.
Secretary and State Health Officer, Florida DOH
1996-1998

In 1992, I had practiced medicine within Florida's public health system for 23 years. At that time, a governmental reorganization, carried out under Governor Lawton Chiles, established the Agency for Healthcare Administration. I was appointed Division Director for Health Policy and Cost Containment in the agency.

The new agency became responsible for a number of non-public health programs that had formerly been administered by the Department of Health and Rehabilitative Services (HRS), including the Florida Medicaid program. HRS was a broad based health and human services department that had been established in 1969. In addition to Medicaid, a number of programs such as Juvenile Justice and Elder Affairs had been removed from the DHRS umbrella. Discussions began about the challenges inherent with public health remaining a part of HRS

Florida's population had been growing rapidly and the decentralized organizational model appeared no longer appropriate to address the continued evolution of health and social issues. The district based structure was not well suited for the highly technical professional disciplines that are essential to public health practice. Although the upper management was dedicated and hard working, the scope and administration of the multiple programs ultimately were proven to be, at best, marginally manageable.

The legislative leaders who were especially dedicated to health and human services included Representative Fred Lippman (D-Broward), Senator Jim King (R-Duval), and William "Doc" Myers (R-Martin). After serious consideration they, and others, reached the conclusion that dividing HRS into two agencies would enable health and social service needs to be met more efficiently. These men were the legislative "fathers" of the new and separate Department of Health. Strong support and active advocacy was provided by Alvin E. Smith, M.D., President of the Florida Medical Association and E. Russell Jackson, Jr., M.A, M.P.H., Senior Vice-President of the Florida Medical Association. The implementing legislation that established the department passed the Florida Senate and House of Representatives unanimously in 1996 with strong bipartisan support. I had been encouraged by the Florida Medical Association to apply for the position of Secretary of the new department and subsequently was appointed by Governor Chiles.

Then came the challenge and excitement of actually building a strong, resilient and effective structure that would allow the growing population's public health needs to be addressed in a comprehensive manner. The executive team along with the public health family worked strenuously to do so. Much credit must be given to Leslie Beitsch, M.D., J.D., Kandy Hill, R.N., B.S., M.S., Richard Hunter, Ph.D. and Wayne McDaniel, M.P.A. for their commitment and dedication. Everyone who worked so hard at this time can be proud of the outcome. A strong infrastructure had been laid by the conclusion of Governor Chiles' second term at the end of 1998. Bipartisan support from the legislature resulted in additional funding for the infrastructure and personnel that were essential to this foundation. The Department of Health was built upon Florida's unique county health department structure. I was pleased to be able to present an excellent Department of Health to the new governor, Jeb Bush, and to the second secretary of the department, Robert Brooks, M.D., M.P.H. ☼

Dr. Howell earned his Bachelor of Science degree from St. John's University in New York in 1962 and his Doctor of Medicine degree from the New York Medical College in 1966. Following an internship, he served as Captain in the Medical Services Corps of the United States Army and Chief of the Preventative Medical Division at Fort Sill, Oklahoma.

After completing a preventive medicine residency in Palm Beach County, Dr. Howell earned a Masters degree from the Harvard School of Public Health and completed the program for Senior Executives in State and Local Government at the John F. Kennedy School of Government at Harvard. He has served in numerous public health positions in Florida, including that of State Health Officer and Secretary of the Florida Department of Health.

Dr. Howell joined the faculty at Nova Southeastern University College of Osteopathic Medicine as Chair of the Department of Rural Medicine in 1999. He is also an Assistant Dean for Professional Relations and a Professor of Public Health.

Dr. Howell played a key role in the founding of the Center for Bioterrorism and All-Hazards Preparedness at Nova Southeastern University. The Center was recognized as one of five national centers funded in part by the Health Resources Services Administration (HRSA) and the U.S. Department of Health and Human Services (DHHS).

In 2009, Dr. Howell was selected as the recipient of the South Florida Business Journal's Excellence in Health Care Awards Lifetime Achievement award.

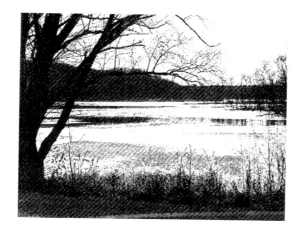

Reflections

Robert G. Brooks, M.D.
Secretary, Florida Department of Health
and State Health Officer
January, 1999 – August, 2001

In November of 1998 the people of Florida elected Jeb Bush as their 43rd Governor. At that time, I was serving in the Florida House of Representatives, and was honored to receive a call from the new Governor. He asked me to be the second Secretary of the Department of Health (DOH). As I reflect on my time served as Secretary, I am reminded most vividly of two vital components to ensuring the protection of the public and the success of the Department: the importance of a strong public health infrastructure, and the critical necessity of a trained and experienced public health workforce.

Early in my tenure as Secretary, we were faced with traditional public health issues and with simultaneously learning to handle more modern problems confronting the field of public health in the nascent 21st century. The combination of traditional and new challenges placed an increasing burden on the shoulders of the DOH leadership and staff.

When I consider traditional public health, I reflect on the ongoing challenges of dealing first with acute, infectious diseases that left unattended can quickly attack the populace with a vengeance. Vaccine-preventable childhood diseases, sexually-transmitted diseases of adolescents and adults, and tuberculosis, come immediately to mind. But many other infections continue to pose major threats as well. For example, shortly after I became Secretary, we were faced with an outbreak of meningococcal meningitis in Putnam County. After epidemiological assessment, it was advised that a mass vaccination campaign should be immediately conducted. This required a team-based approach that was effectively carried out to limit the spread of this deadly disease. Also, while other outbreaks of traditional infections occurred during those years, none probably was more defining than the discovery of West Nile virus in Florida beginning in the summer of 2001. Because of a state-of-the-art virology lab, backed up by sound epidemiological support, we were able to identify this emerging pathogen early in its introduction into the state, initiate a plan of interdiction, and minimize human cases – a testament to a well-functioning public health team!

While public health will continue to have to deal with the acute, infectious agents that have defined this field for centuries, the last 30 years have brought new challenges to public health through the need to treat chronic diseases of health importance as well. As far back as the 1960s and 70s, public health began to be involved with programs to deal with new diseases attendant to life-style choices. At first there was smoking, then obesity, and subsequently HIV/AIDS- all resulting in major public health problems of chronic duration.

When I arrived in January of 1999, the Department had already begun the first full year of funding for tobacco education and interdiction. Tens of millions of dollars were poured into a broad, exciting initiative to assure that Floridians- particularly teens and pre-teens, knew about the public health hazards of first-hand and second-hand smoke. Over the course of the first legislative session, our unusual challenge was to convince the legislature the DOH could put into place an evidence-based program that would spend appropriated dollars for maximum effectiveness. In later years this program, unfortunately, saw significant changes in funding but, the Truth Campaign was able – through the hard work of so many DOH employees, to keep thousands of teens off of tobacco.

In addition to the traditional infectious and preventable diseases of public health, and the new chronic diseases needing attention, a third area of public health challenge became evident: disaster preparedness. While the atrocities of 9/11 and subsequent anthrax were to occur later, the state already had its own share of natural disasters that required a prepared public health workforce. In 1999, we were tested by the massive storm known now as Hurricane Floyd. While Florida was spared the major devastation of this storm as it turned at the last minute from hitting our east coast, to subsequently impact further north, it tested our readiness and prepared us for the major hurricanes of 2004 and 2005.

I would also call attention to several other important events defining this period of time in the Florida DOH. First, was the attention to quality improvement. Under the leadership particularly of Les Beitsch and Kathy Mason, the QI team made the Florida DOH a national leader in public health QI and an early candidate for accreditation. Second, was a focus on health disparities. Thanks to the leadership of Governor Bush, we were able to start the "Closing the Gap" grant program to work with community-based organizations on six key health disparities in the minority population. Third, was an emphasis on the importance of the local health department in the success of public health. During my term I was able to visit all 67 counties in Florida- every health department at least once. Everywhere I went I found the same high caliber of people who were dedicating their lives to help others through their work in public health at the local (and in some cases state and national) level.

Reflecting on these years at the Department of Health there are certainly many other accomplishments that the staff can be proud of, but none of them could have been attained without a team of dedicated public health individuals at all levels. As Secretary, I know my work was made possible only because of the expertise and, at times, sacrifices of many others. I would particularly thank the Deputy Secretaries that served with me including, Les Beitsch, Rick

Hunter, Wayne McDaniel, Eric Handler, and John Agwunobi. Their dedication to the work of promoting and protecting the health of the people of this state was exemplary. ☀

Dr. Brooks is the Associate Dean for Health Affairs and Professor of Family Medicine and Rural Health at the Florida State University College of Medicine. He received his B.A. and M.D. degrees from Wayne State University in Detroit, and is Board-certified in Internal Medicine and Infectious Diseases. He practiced medicine from 1984 through 1999 in Orlando, Florida, during which time he served as Assistant Director of the Internal Medicine Residency Program and Chief of Infectious Diseases at the Orlando Regional Medical Center. In November of 1994, Dr. Brooks was elected to the Florida House of Representatives where he served until appointed Secretary of the Florida Department of Health by then newly-elected Governor Jeb Bush in late 1998. In September of 2001, Dr. Brooks joined the academic team at Florida State University involved with establishing the first new allopathic medical school in the U.S. in over 20 years. Since joining the medical school he has established four separate Centers of Excellence, including Centers on Terrorism and Public Health, Patient Safety, Rural Health, and Medicine and Public Health.

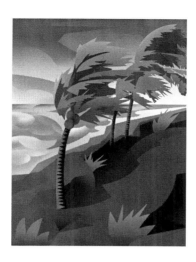

Heroes

John Agwunobi MD MBA MPH
Secretary of the Department of Health
2001-2004

My tenure as Secretary of Health was one marked by the Attack on the World Trade Center on 9/11, the Anthrax attack in Boca Raton in October 2001, Bioterrorism response, West Nile Virus, Hurricanes, and so much more. But the one thing that held true across all these events and the many others that we had to deal with as a team, was the passion, skill, self-sacrifice and commitment of the Florida Public Health professional that I served alongside. In December 2002, while serving as the Secretary of the Florida Department of Health, I wrote an editorial that was published in the Tallahassee Democrat in early January 2003; it included the following excerpt...

If you were asked to nominate someone for "Floridian of the Year," whom would you select? If I were ever asked to choose, it would be a soldier of sorts, yet no less a warrior. Invisible to most, a stranger to many, my choice battled valiantly all year long to promote and protect the health and safety of everyone in Florida. My nominee would be the great Florida public health professional.

The fine men and women who make up this dedicated corps of public servants have long deserved but rarely received our collective recognition for their hard work. Recent years have overflowed with unprecedented public health challenges but through it all, Florida's public health professionals stood tall. Public health responded to many environmental health hazards this year. Whether fecal bacteria in the sea, dioxin in fish or arsenic in wells, these professionals threw themselves into the fray with an enthusiasm born of their desire to save lives.

Today, Florida breathes easier in the knowledge that its public health professionals displayed excellence and dedication in their response to the very real threats posed by the SARS and influenza outbreaks of 2003. The ubiquitous mosquito provided a number of opportunities for public health to prove its mettle this year. At all points on the Florida compass, our public health crew helped the state navigate through seasonal squalls of West Nile Virus and Eastern Equine Encephalitis. In South Florida, malaria reared its ugly head, only to have it decapitated by the very capable Palm Beach public health battalion.

Even as hordes of mosquitoes tried to inject us with their deadly diseases, swarms of public health professionals inoculated thousands of their fellow Floridians against smallpox, meningitis, influenza and hepatitis. In this new world of weapons of mass destruction and bioterrorism, we have come to appreciate that public health is our weapon of mass defense. Public health sentinels line the ramparts of our homeland, alert and poised to respond.

Today, few states can claim to have as finely prepared a public health army as that which endows Florida. In the face of such an extraordinary year, many wrongly expected our public health professionals to waiver in their commitment to basic public health services. Whether it was tobacco use, obesity or HIV/AIDS, public health professionals redoubled their efforts to reduce the number affected or at risk. They continued to deliver comprehensive refugee health services to our newest Floridians while ensuring access to primary health care for our poorest Floridians.

To my nominee for "Floridian of the year": For your excellence, commitment and hard work promoting and protecting health and safety in Florida throughout 2003, I salute you.

Even today as I re-read this Op Ed I realize it was a singularly amazing time. My most prominent memories are those that reflect the nature, the metal, the character of the Florida Public Health professional, the men and women who even today, tirelessly do battle for the health of their fellow citizens in Florida. As I recall, 2003 went on to be an extremely busy public health year but by some accounts the year that followed, 2004, was our finest. That was the year Florida was hit by four major hurricanes within weeks of each other. In our time of greatest need, our Public Health team stood up once again and proved to the world why the Florida Department of Health was the jewel of government and a model of service.

I remember every storm as if it was yesterday but our response to the last storm, Hurricane Ivan, jumps to mind, as I reflect, especially our effort to relieve our fellow workers from a crowded and overwhelmed hurricane medical relief shelter in Pensacola in the days that followed.

We decided it was imperative to take supplies and a team of nurses to Pensacola to relieve the crew that had manned the hurricane shelter in the Pensacola Community College gymnasium for the two days that straddled the coming ashore of Hurricane Ivan. We had gotten word that they were straining under the workload and the dire conditions of the aftermath of the storm.

We gathered in the small airport lobby that early morning. As the glass doors opened we were hit with a blast of hot humid air from the tarmac outside. We stepped out into the ferocious Tallahassee sun and walked the 100 yards to the National Guard helicopter that awaited us. The Chinook helicopter was so much bigger in real life than it looked in pictures and movies.

As we boarded the ramp in the rear I had to let my eyes adjust to the abrupt change from the bright sun outside to the dim light of the cavernous belly of the bi-rotor beast. I could see that each wall was lined by hammock type seating made from webbing. Strapped into each seat was one of almost fifty nurses. All had volunteered from County Health Departments across North Florida to go to Pensacola to help relieve their colleagues in the shelter. No one talked on the one hour flight. The noise of the rotors was deafening and everyone was overcome with the enormity of the event and the work to come. As they clutched their backpacks and duffle bags tightly their faces expressed nervous anticipation and excitement. Only a couple had ever flown in a helicopter before and many had not practiced clinical nursing in years but they volunteered anyway.

We landed outside of the Pensacola and boarded military trucks to the College. Pensacola felt like a war zone. Almost two full days after the storm and even with a police escort the trip was treacherous as we swerved around tree limbs downed street signs and traffic lights, power lines and other hurricane debris. The city had taken a pounding. The only folks out on the streets appeared to be National Guard officers helping man intersections. The parking lot of the college was filled with parked cars many damaged by debris that had blown in on Hurricane Ivan. Many had dents and broken windows. Pebbles used to coat the flat roofs of the surrounding buildings had been blown of the roof and fired at more than 130 miles per hour across the parking lot like a hailstorm of bullets.

The gymnasium was packed with people on cots, and on blankets on the floor. The sounds and smells will stay with me forever. The nurses that had opened and manned the shelter had not been home since the day before the storm hit. Many did not know if their family and homes had weathered the storm as cell phone coverage was lost in the hours that followed. They were exhausted physically and mentally drained but not one of them left till they transitioned the hundreds of fragile, sick and elderly citizens under their care, to the relief team. I have never been more moved by the selfless sacrifice and compassion of a dedicated group of professionals than on that day.

As I think back on my days in the Florida Department of Health the story above is one of a thousand stories that remind me of how lucky and privileged I was to serve alongside each and every one of the public health workers who worked in every county health department, headquarters and outpost of the Florida Health Department. Each and everyone is a hero in my mind. ⚜

Dr. John O. Agwunobi, as senior vice president and president of health and wellness for Walmart US, oversees the company's health and wellness business unit, including pharmacies, vision centers and health care clinics. He joined the company in September 2007.

Prior to joining Walmart, he was the Assistant Secretary for Health for the U.S. Department of Health and Human Services and an Admiral in the U.S. Public Health Service Commissioned Corps. In that role he was responsible for overseeing the US Public Health Service including the CDC, NIH, FDA, SAMSA, Indian Health Services and the Office of the US Surgeon General. Before this position, Dr. Agwunobi served from October 2001 to September 2005 as Florida's Secretary of Health, reporting to Governor Jeb Bush. Dr. Agwunobi, a pediatrician, previously served as vice president of a pediatric rehabilitation hospital and medical director for an affiliated managed care plan in Washington, D.C.

Dr. Agwunobi attended medical school at the University of Jos in Nigeria. He completed residency training in pediatrics at Howard University in Washington DC. He did his Masters in Business Administration (MBA) at Georgetown in Washington DC and his Masters in Public Health at Johns Hopkins School of Public Health in Baltimore.

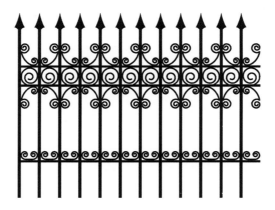

Breaking Barriers

By M. Rony Francois, MD, MSPH, PhD
Secretary, Florida Department of Health
2005-2007

The message was brief, but incredulous and life-changing. On a warm Friday afternoon in August 2005, I received a phone call from Mr. Mark Kaplan, then Governor Jeb Bush's Chief of Staff. The Governor had appointed me as Secretary of the Florida Department of Health!

My experience thus far had been in academia at the University of South Florida, College of Public Health, where I was directing the Public Health Practice Program, a distance learning Master's in Public Health Program for health professionals. I had also been serving as a site Medical Director for CHD Meridian at Citigroup in Tampa. This call to public service gave me the unexpected privilege of following into the honorable footsteps of Andre G. Francois, my departed Dad, who had served with distinction and integrity as Undersecretary of Interior in Haiti.

The special day of my historical appointment announcement came quickly as Governor Bush welcomed and introduced me as the first Haitian-American to lead a state agency. In my acceptance speech, I thanked the Governor and noted my remarkable return to Tallahassee where I had begun my educational journey 25 years earlier at Tallahassee Community College. I expressed my vision to fulfill the noble mission of the department, which is **to promote and protect the health of all the citizens of our beloved state.**

- I highlighted the word "**all**" to emphasize our collective duty to provide competent, just, and compassionate care in a totally inclusive fashion.
- I underscored the word "**promote**," which implies that preventive strategies must become an integral part of health care.
- I emphasized the word "**protect**" and renewed our commitment to health and safety for all Floridians.
- I singled out the word "**health**" and reminded our patients and clients that health is not simply the absence of disease, but a state where stress management, good nutrition, and regular exercise allow the attainment of wellness. And, the Romans said it best: "Mens sana in corpore sano"; or, "a healthy mind in a healthy body!"

Finally, I expressed a prophetic word of caution about public health's standing in government and reminded the audience that Hurricane Katrina's recent fury and devastation had taught us many lessons. My hope was that in the near future, public health's critical role in our daily lives would be fully recognized without the sinister help of a natural or man-made catastrophe.

During my fifteen-month tenure as the Secretary of Health and State Health Officer for the State of Florida, I knew that leadership, even with an agenda of continuity, first required the establishment of a respectful and direct human connection with as many staff as possible. I traveled over 68,000 miles on state business in that short period, visiting County Health Departments where I was privileged to learn in some instances that I was the first Secretary to visit the premises.

Once trust was established with my team, we had many firsts:

- We developed the first ever strategic plan for the entire Department as well as for public health preparedness.
- We established the first Inter-Agency Collaboration focusing on Women's Health issues and held the first Annual Women's Health

Conference. At that time, Florida was one of only four states with a strategic plan specific for improving women's health.

- We developed a Burn Care protocol and training program for Trauma Centers that have been adopted as the national model by the U.S. Department of Health & Human Services, the U.S. Health Resources Administration, the American College of Surgeons, and the American Burn Association.
- Our Team convened the first statewide meeting of the Nursing Leadership in Florida (Private sector, government, and academia) to address workforce shortages and other issues.
- Although an Office of Minority Health had statutorily been established, the position had not been filled. So, I made this search a priority and recruited the very first Minority Health Director in the history of the state of Florida to address health disparities in the sunshine state.

Setting direction in a large organization may also require substantive change. The following leadership challenge illustrates my ability to deal with critical situations and to bring the necessary organizational metamorphosis, in spite of political pressures. In this example, I had to weigh healthcare practitioners' ability to practice versus the safety of the public. I concluded that practicing one's health profession is not a right but a privilege that can be taken away if the care cannot be given safely. While Florida's Health Secretary, I suspended hundreds of healthcare practitioners' licenses for infractions ranging from fraud, standards of practice issues, to substance abuse. With respect to the latter, I quickly recognized that the cases were taking several years to get to my desk. The providers involved would just be given another treatment contract, in spite of repeated therapeutic compliance violations, such as positive drug screens, missed counseling sessions, and would essentially be allowed to continue to practice in spite of their uncontrolled impairment. In many of these provider impairment cases, patients were sexually abused, narcotics were repeatedly diverted from vulnerable patients, and standards of practice were not followed.

The nurses enrolled in the Intervention Project for Nurses (IPN) had a different set of rules than the doctors being treated by the

Professionals Resource Network (PRN), a subsidiary of the Florida Medical Association (FMA). So, I called the Medical Directors of the two treatment programs into my office. They were agency contractors and I requested that the critical services provided by both IPN and PRN be improved.

The FMA, who controls the PRN treatment program and the Florida Board of Medicine wrote to the Governor and challenged my actions. As an occupational medicine specialist, I knew that we had stricter drug testing and treatment compliance guidelines for the bus drivers who operate our school buses. Indeed, if they have one positive drug screen, they are out of a job and it does not take 3-7 years. In spite of the FMA's challenges, I pursued the needed changes. As a result, new guidelines for the treatment programs emerged. The details of these new policies were actually developed by IPN and PRN with some oversight from the Department. Today, the impaired practitioner programs for both Nurses (Intervention Project for Nurses) and physicians (PRN) are better and stronger than before. Because of the improvements I triggered, the problematic rules that had been in place for about 25 years in the State of Florida were revamped and are now the same for all healthcare practitioners. If they violate their substance abuse treatment contract 3 times, the Board is notified and action is taken, such as voluntary relinquishment of their license. Criminal actions are now immediately reported to law enforcement and are no longer protected by one's treatment status.

In my role as the State Health Officer, I embraced and supported the noble mission of safeguarding the health and safety of the entire population. Our teams of professionals applied the most effective interventions in order to reduce morbidity and mortality. We monitored program accomplishments closely. However, changing individual's behaviors in order to achieve collective success which was measured by increasing rates of immunizations, decreasing Sexually Transmitted Disease rates, lowering infant mortality, reducing obesity rates was our biggest challenge.

We worked tirelessly to make a difference. Examples of our successes include:
- Immunization rates for two-year olds reached 2nd highest in the nation
- Perinatally-acquired HIV cases reduced from 172 to 5

- Developed a comprehensive Pandemic influenza plan for Florida in preparation for possible epidemic including an ethics component
- Florida cancer data system attained "Gold Standard Award" for 3rd year in a row
- Decreased the prevalence rate of current cigarette use by 60 percent among middle school students and by 42.7 percent among high school students and smoking prevalence among Florida's adult smokers decreased from 22 percent to 17.3 percent over eight years.
- AG Holley State Hospital achieved a 93% cure rate on most difficult tuberculosis cases vs. traditional cure rate of 50%
- Trained more than 1,000 laboratory workers on chemical terrorism and all 5 public health labs have biosafety level 3 capacity
- Initiated real time "paperless" electronic public health disease reporting for laboratories
- Held inaugural summit, "Meeting of the Minds, Research for New Insights and Innovative Cures" in 2006 to develop a statewide research agenda to expedite funding cures for the most deadly diseases.
- Met Healthy People 2010 Goals related to diabetes screening
- First successful initiatives to empower youth as ambassadors for promoting healthy behaviors and coordinating physical activities in their schools and communities.
- Promoted statewide health and wellness campaign (Step-Up Florida) in all 67 counties in Florida to encourage policy and environmental changes to increase healthy behaviors (installation of walking trails and healthy choices in school vending machines).
- Commissioned the Drowning Prevention Pilot Study to raise awareness for the prevention of drowning in the 0-4 age group for which Florida has the highest rates in the nation. We cultivated unique community partnerships and worked with Denny's restaurants to distribute 800,000 interactive water safety materials and prevention messages on drowning in Florida and held multiple local awareness campaign events in about a dozen cities in the state.

I have often said, "In any organization, the services provided are only as good as the people who provide them." Consequently, workforce development was made a priority. The goal of that process was to develop trusting relationships by demonstrating an empathetic commitment to staff development on multiple levels. The first level focused on encouraging professional growth through the pursuit of educational opportunities such as online certificates, degrees, workshops, training, and conferences. The second aspect dealt with succession planning. Because we had an aging workforce in public health, it was critical that our most senior staff mentor and nurture the next generation so that there was no interruption in the services we provided upon their retirement. The last level called for public health professionals to model the practice of healthy lifestyles that we preach: nutritious diet, regular physical activity, and effective stress management. Practicing these habits ourselves increased our ability to change others' behaviors and also improved our staff's quality of life.

In terms of vision, I proposed the concept of the Public Health Apprenticeship Program to the Centers for Disease Control and Prevention (CDC). I was aware that at the national level a pipeline for public health professionals was absent with the exception of epidemiologists. A CDC Senior Management Official approached me about submitting one project idea to the CDC. Aware of our aging workforce in public health, I immediately expressed the desire to develop a formal entry-level apprenticeship program for the nation. I also shared my vision and approach for a sound framework that would assure the development of our future national public health workforce. As a result of this effort, the CDC received over 1400 applications for the Public Health Apprenticeship Program in 2010. This year's class of 65 apprentices will be training in 27 states.

Finally, I am pleased to note that I had the privilege of interacting with foreign government officials as I traveled internationally as Florida's Health Secretary five times. I visited the Bahamas (4th Caribbean Regional Chiefs of Mission Conference on HIV/AIDS and one Public Health Mission), Haiti (Presidential US Delegation and one Public Health Mission), and the Dominican Republic (one Public Health Mission). The three public health missions aimed at providing technical assistance and distance learning opportunities on emergency preparedness and on public health to our neighboring ministries of health.

As we tackle our current health challenges across the country, I believe that we ought to look beyond our borders, since best practices transcend man-made frontiers. Consequently, as we provide other nations with requested technical assistance, we need to approach these opportunities with the humility necessary to recognize and bring back effective interventions to the U.S.

Our accomplishments during my tenure could not have been possible without the unwavering perseverance of our Staff at the local, county, and state levels. I was indeed blessed to work with a talented group whom I supported tirelessly. I applaud the entire public health team in Florida as I am certain that their selfless dedication and professionalism will continue to make a daily difference in the lives of Floridians for years to come.

Finally, I share my own guiding principle: "Salve populi, suprema lex!" or "The safeguard of the people (is, ought to be), the supreme law (of the land)!" ☼

M. Rony François, M.D., MA, M.S.P.H., Ph.D., is currently a Courtesy Affiliate Assistant Professor at the USF Colleges of Medicine and Public Health. Dr. Francois is the immediate past State Health Officer and Director of the Division of Public Health (DPH) for the Georgia Department of Community Health (DCH). Dr. François oversaw programs responsible for disease control and prevention and the promotion of healthy lifestyles. Prior to joining DCH, Dr. François served as the Assistant Secretary for the Office of Public Health at the Louisiana Department of Health and Hospitals where he was responsible for the direction and management of the state's public health programs with a budget of about $330M. Under his leadership in 2009, the Louisiana Immunization Program was ranked second in the nation by the Centers for Disease Control and Prevention (CDC). Dr. Francois is also the immediate past Secretary of Health and State Health Officer for the State of Florida where he was instrumental with agency accomplishments such as having the second highest immunization rate in the nation for two-year olds. Dr. François brings perspectives from academia and the private sector. He was an Assistant Professor and Director of the Public Health Practice Program at the University Of South Florida College Of Public Health, and worked as the Site Medical Director for Corporate Health Dimensions at Citigroup in Tampa for over seven years.

With an extensive academic background including a Master of Arts in Exercise Physiology from the University of Central Florida (UCF), a Doctor of Medicine degree, a Master of Science in Public Health, and a Doctor of Philosophy in Toxicology/Public Health degree from the University of South Florida, Dr. François is passionate about the public's health and is a strong advocate for providing quality health services for all. Fluent in French, Creole, and limited Spanish, Dr. François is also an inventor. He has worked as a teacher, cardiac rehabilitation exercise physiologist, and has played professional soccer. He was named All-American in 1982 and inducted into the UCF Athletics Hall of Fame in 2005 for his accomplishments in soccer.

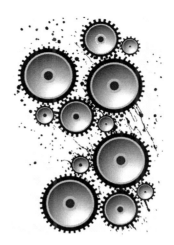

Come Together

By Ana Maria Viamonte Ros, MD, MPH
Secretary, Department of Health & State Surgeon General
January 2007- January 2011

As State Surgeon General, there were three defining events that I will never forget; the earthquake in Haiti and subsequent cholera epidemic, H1N1 flu and the oil spill in the Gulf of Mexico. These tragedies garnered national and international attention. The collaborative response specific to each of these events is what resonates with me. Witnessing the dedication of state and local health officials, federal agencies, academic institutions, community partners, not-for-profit organizations and Florida residents affirms my belief that through collaboration, anything can be accomplished.

I traveled as a member of a medical mission to several developing nations and had just traveled to Haiti, the poorest country in the western hemisphere and one of the least developed, the week of Thanksgiving 2009. I was devastated when I heard of the 7.0 magnitude earthquake that struck Haiti in the afternoon of January 12, 2010. The epicenter was located near the town of Leogane, approximately 16 miles west of Port Au Prince, but the destruction was far-reaching and the ongoing aftershocks that occurred for days compounded the damage. This earthquake was the 6th deadliest ever recorded. While casualty numbers may never be known, approximately 230,000 people died, approximately 300,000 people were injured, and more than 1.5 million people became homeless in a matter of minutes.

Following the earthquake, the Department of Health worked closely with our state and federal partners to provide assistance and support to the response teams of health care providers and search and rescue personnel who departed for Haiti. We also provided assistance to those who came to Florida on repatriation flights or as humanitarian medical evacuees. Florida did not turn away any survivors in need of medical treatment. Nearly 7,000 patients were received from medical evacuation or repatriation flights and treated; more than 600 were hospitalized for extended care and treatment. Our personnel worked tirelessly to meet the needs of every person, from those with the most critical injuries to those who accompanied them without physical ills but suffering from mental anguish.

I was impressed with the way our health and emergency response communities came together to support the people of Haiti during the aftermath of this catastrophic event. The sites I saw in the aftermath of the earthquake created memories that I will never forget.

Our efforts in assisting our Haitian neighbors occurred while we were already in the process of executing an ambitious H1N1 influenza vaccination campaign. This campaign helped not only reduce H1N1 disease, but our coordinated public and private sector efforts have also reduced the burden on our health care systems. Florida's H1N1 efforts were supported by an aggressive disease surveillance program that aimed to ensure both the health care community and the public received up-to-date information.

The campaign was incredibly successful! Together, we immunized over 2.1 million Floridians with the help of more than 4,700 providers at more than 5,000 sites. Vaccine sites included doctor's offices, hospitals, walk-in clinics, county health departments and pharmacies throughout the state. Further, my quoting of 4,700 providers is a conservative estimate because, in many instances, one registered provider represented at least two or three other providers in the same the medical facility. Amassing a statewide team was critical to keeping the spread and impact of H1N1 at bay—even still, over 1,200 Floridians were hospitalized because of H1N1, and millions more were affected.

The explosion of the Deepwater Horizon drilling rig and subsequent months of spilling oil was another disaster that affected millions of Floridians, as well as our neighbors along the Gulf Coast. Florida was fortunate that the oil spill did not reach our shores until June 4, 2010. This triggered our response phase.

Again, we were privileged that Florida has a mature and experienced emergency management system. Under the leadership of Governor Charlie Crist, the State Emergency Response Team, of which DOH is a member, and the Florida Department of Environmental Protection coordinated and simultaneously responded to the impacts from the Deepwater Horizon incident. Many Florida officials, including myself, remain deeply concerned about the long-term impacts from the Deepwater Horizon oil spill on our state's economy, coastal tourism, environment, wildlife, and of course, the health and wellbeing of our residents and those who assisted with the clean-up efforts.

While I write at length about these events, I'd be remiss not to mention the other long-term challenges to the health of Floridians like tobacco use and overweight and obesity rates, particularly among our youth. The Florida Department of Health as an agency also faces challenges—most notably another budget shortfall as the state begins planning for the 2011-12 fiscal year.

As Florida's first Surgeon General, I feel honored to have worked and collaborated with such a dedicated team of public health professionals. ☀

Dr. Viamonte-Ros earned her medical degree from the University of Miami School of Medicine and her Masters of Public Health degree from Harvard. She was the first Florida Surgeon General where she headed Florida's $3 billion Department of Health, with a staff of 17,000 and 300 sites in 67 counties. She also developed 11 pilot sites, as part of Florida's first healthcare reform initiative. She recently joined the staff of Health Resources, Ltd. as Vice President of Development and Public Affairs.

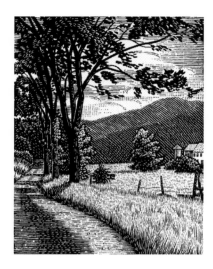

The Road Less Traveled:
Carl L. Brumback, MD

From the Florida Medical Association

W hen Carl L. Brumback, MD, graduated from medical school, he could not have known where his life would lead. He quickly became accustomed to taking the road less traveled, forging new paths that today remain vital to public health in Florida. From the halls of Alcatraz to the rubble of post-war Germany, Dr. Brumback's life ultimately led him to Palm Beach County. There, working to improve the lives of the public including indigent migrant workers, he founded a health department that now stands as a model for the nation. Dr. Brumback's great passion for health care and can-do spirit continue to positively affect the lives of others, leaving a legacy that only grows stronger with time.

A Life Less Ordinary

After receiving his medical degree from the University of Kansas School of Medicine, Brumback headed west to pursue a residency in San Francisco, beginning his career in a United States Marine Hospital. During this period, nearby Alcatraz Island still was housing some of America's most dangerous criminals. Only two physicians worked in the infirmary, and when one of them became ill and had to retire, the marine hospital began rotating residents. "My wife, Lucile, would take me to the pier. She was a real partner to me." Dr. Brumback remembers. "Prison workers picked me up in a boat and took me to the island. Then two guards escorted me through six gates to the infirmary and physician's office." During a shift, Brumback would conduct rounds along "Broadway," the cell block corridor, examining prisoners under the watchful eye of armed guards. During this time, he examined crime figures such as Robert "Machine Gun" Kelly, a notable prohibition-era gangster, and Robert Franklin Stroud, better known as the "Birdman of Alcatraz."

After Brumback worked in San Francisco, he served as a physician in the United States Army in Europe where World War II turned in favor of the Allies, leading ultimately to victory. As a result, the United States Army began discharging soldiers. Unfortunately, they discharged far more physicians than necessary and created a shortage in war-torn Germany. "There were ships sunk all over the harbor," he says. "They loaded us on a train into what they called forty-and-eight cars, because they could hold either forty men or eight horses." The train stopped in Cassel, Germany, where Brumback would take post as Deputy Commander of a military hospital. "Cassel was pretty well pulverized," he says. "There were only a few buildings intact along the outskirts." One of these buildings had served as headquarters to Hitler's Western Commander, who had vacated his office so hastily that he left his epaulets and Nazi insignia behind in their display case. "The hospital commander chose to leave them where they were," says Brumback. "They ended up being quite the conversation piece."

After 16 months in Europe, Brumback returned to the United States and decided to pursue additional post-graduate work at the University of Michigan. There, he received a Master of Public Health degree and developed a passionate interest in providing care to underserved communities. His desire was simple: he wanted to combine the efforts of the public and private sectors, increasing the level of cooperation between physicians and public health workers to create a better system of care. Members of the Michigan faculty alerted Brumback to an opportunity in Oak Ridge, Tennessee, at the Atomic Energy Commission. A Michigan professor was on his way there to aid in reorganizing the health system and Brumback was invited to join him. After a few months in Tennessee, the two men achieved great results and Brumback became the director of the project. Yet, he felt compelled to move on. "I wanted to get out of federal service," says Brumback. "I wanted to get into communities to address health problems affecting people in genuine need."

Aware of Dr. Brumback's work at the Atomic Energy Commission, Florida State Health Officer, Wilson T. Sowder, M.D. recommended him to create a county health department in Palm Beach. "I told him I wanted to tackle every conceivable health problem and develop the resources to do so. He told me this was just the place I was looking for."

From the Ground Up

Soon after arriving, Brumback became involved in organized medicine. He joined the Florida Medical Association (FMA) and also the Palm Beach County Medical Society (PBCMS). Before taking his post at the health department, the PBCMS assembled a committee of physician leadership to interview him. "They wanted to know what my plan was," says Brumback. "I told them that I didn't have one, but I committed to them that we would work together to identify the county's health problems and to identify solutions." Dr. Brumback and the physicians of Palm Beach County were quickly on the same page. He soon became a member of the Palm Beach County Medical Society's Executive Committee and thus began a journey toward building one of the finest public health systems in the country, which has as its foundation a strong partnership between public health and the private practice of medicine.

The immediate challenges were overwhelming. "When I took over as director of the health department in 1950, there were 114,000 residents in the county, and I had a budget of $92,000," Brumback says. To make matters worse, Palm Beach County had one of the largest populations of migrant farm workers in the nation – roughly 55,000. "There were very few physicians in the area at the time an even fewer specialists. By the time many of the emigrant workers received medical attention, their cases were terminal." Their living conditions were abysmal; making homes out of packing crates in spares labor camps.

Dr. Brumback began taking photographs, documenting the misfortune of the emigrant workers. He contacted groups like the Florida Christian Migrant Ministry and organized efforts to raise awareness, funding, and cooperative action. This led him as far as Washington, D.C., where he gave a presentation to a national council of churches and ministries, sharing his photographs and eyewitness accounts of the problem. Although he had no trouble stirring interest in solving the problem, funding was another story.

Then, in 1954, Brumback received a federal grant to study the health of migrant workers that resulted in a book by the study's principal investigator, Earl L. Koos, PhD, head of the Department of Social Anthropology at Florid State University. The book, titled, *They Follow the Sun*, further documented Florida's struggling population of migrant workers. The two men began communicating and sharing ideas.

"Dr. Koos understood that addressing the problem would require more than medical care." says Brumback. "These people needed aid in every conceivable way, and providing it would require a team effort among physicians, educators, and public health workers."

Dr. Brumback and Dr. Koos approached Elisabeth Peabody, MD, a pediatrician with the United States Children's Bureau, about funding a project. "The woman was a magician," says Brumback, laughing. "She came up with $250,000 to see what our proposed team could do in Palm Beach County." The team would use two new health centers in Belle Glade to treat migrant workers and their families and ultimately attract attention from Washington. Dr. Brumback's program became a national model, the inspiration for a multi-million dollar federal program to build similar migrant health programs throughout the United States. In 1962, Brumback was appointed as a member of a national committee responsible for supervision these programs to ensure their success.

Uncharted Territory

As Brumback fought to improve the lives of migrant workers, he still had a county health department to run. Unfortunately, with limited funding, he had very few obvious resources. "I knew I needed an assistant," he says, "but I did not have the money to afford the quality of physician I needed." This gave Brumback an idea. Rather than looking for experienced physicians at a discount, he developed a residency program, looking to attract talented young graduates form the nation's top medical schools. "It was a strange idea," says Brumback. "Health departments did not house residencies." Nonetheless, he wrote the national accrediting board and was approved. One of his first residents, James T. Howell, MD, would go on to become the first Secretary of the Florida Department of Health. Another, Jean M. Malecki, MD, now serves as Director of the Palm Beach County Health Department. Under her guidance the department has grown rapidly, employing hundreds, with a budget of nearly $70 million. Their residency program continues to attract top young physicians from all over the world.

Many of the groundbreaking programs Dr. Brumback developed over the years in Palm Beach County remain active and have been duplicated by other county departments across Florida. He developed an Environmental Health and Engineering Department to monitor all aspects of air, water and land pollution. "When I came back in 1950, Palm Beach County had a considerable pollution problem. They didn't have sewage processing, so we organized a system to deliver it and the standards to enforce it."

Every step of the way, Brumback worked to involve private physicians in public matters. Unfortunately, state laws at the time did not permit general medical care in county health departments. Impressed by his successes in aiding the migrant population in Palm beach, a West Palm Beach City commissioner approached Brumback about developing similar support systems in the county. "I explained to him that we were limited according to the statutes in term of providing direct medical care," says Brumback. "That kind of program simply did not exist."

The two men traveled to Jacksonville and met with State Health Officer Sowder, explaining their desires. "I can still see him," says Brumback. "I can still hear his voice. He listened to us, then he looked at me and said, 'What you're proposing is the wave of the future.'" Dr. Sowder recommended a waiver from state law, allowing Brumback's efforts to proceed toward revolutionary change for a closer partnership between the public and private sector of health care in Florida.

Wave of the Future

Throughout his career, Dr. Brumback brought "wave of the future" health care of Florida. Serving as Chair of the FMA Public Health Committee, his wisdom, insight and division ensured that Florida's physicians were active in public health decisions throughout the state. He also received innumerable awards and accolades, including the American Medical Association's highest honor: the Dr. Nathan Davis Award. Yet, perhaps the most impressive characteristic of Dr. Brumback's career remains his day-to-day persistence and clear-eyed vision and resilience in navigating uncharted territory and forging new paths.

Even after retiring, Dr. Brumback continued working with the Palm Beach County Health Department Residency Program for fourteen years. Now 95 years of age, Dr. Brumback still lives in Palm Beach Gardens and continues to give lectures promoting the residency program. His goal is to continue the program's tradition of attracting talented young physicians from all over the world. "I only wish more physicians could take advantage of it," says Brumback. Generations of physicians and patients alike have benefited from his contributions to medicine and public health in Florida. It stems from career devoted to creating better opportunities for others and a lifelong commitment to excellence. Today the influence of Carl L. Brumback, MD, is undeniable and his extraordinary legacy continues to grow.

Story Update: We are sorry to say that Dr. Brumback passed away on January 13, 2012 at the age of 97.

Special thanks to the Florida Medical Association for allowing us to republish this article.

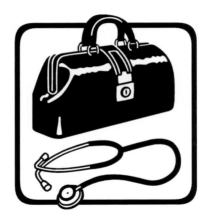

Remembering
Dr. Carl L. Brumback
Palm Beach County
Public Health Director
1914 – 2012

By Alina M. Alonso, M.D.

It was in 1991 on a hot, humid, summer day after a long Fourth of July weekend, that I sat anxiously waiting to hear my first Monday morning lecture from the iconic and renowned Dr. Carl L. Brumback. I was aware of his long, distinguished and intriguing public health career at the Palm Beach County Health Department. Although he retired, he was still volunteering by teaching residents Preventive Medicine/Public Health Residency Program which he personally created back in 1956. I was now one of those physicians. I had not exactly chosen to do this residency out of a desire to further my medical education, but rather at the convincing of Dr. Jean Malecki who was at that time the Director of the County Health Department. She insisted that the future of medicine was not to treat but to prevent diseases. So, I prepared myself by searching for anything I could find about Dr. Brumback from several historical books I found in the library.

I expected to see a tall grey-haired older man make an entrance in a designer suit with shiny shoes. I imagined a lecture full of "glory days in public health" with lots of famous names being dropped as to impress the new residents. I expected to be lectured about all the duties needed to run the largest area health department east of the Mississippi. I even expected him to show us slides of his work out in the migrant camps and how he had solved all the problems in the Glades.

Instead, to my amazement, upon his arrival, he walked slowly but deliberately towards the front of the room. He was much smaller than I had imagined, but there was a presence about him that commanded one's attention and respect. There was no introduction. He pulled up a plastic chair and sat right beside the residents with hand written notes on plain white paper which he held folded through the entire lecture. He never once glanced at his notes. His powder blue blazer matched his eyes as he began with the words, "The one sure thing that you can count on in Public Health is that you will never have enough money or staff to do the things you want to do for your community. When you work in Public Health, you work for your community, not yourself."

As he was reminiscing about public health, he talked about several incidents that changed the course of public health in Palm Beach County, including how he traveled along with a nurse in his Rambler Nash Station Wagon throughout the county to treat migrants and children. He talked about how he set out to enlist nutritionists and social workers to create a wellness program for those migrants. He discussed how during his early years as the Director he made the connection between the pattern of out-pouring of raw sewage into the Intracoastal Waterway and an outbreak of polio. He continued his discussion by sharing his vision to set up a mental health clinic along with medical clinics, as a way to save the taxpayer's money and increase access to care in Palm Beach County. He shared how he supported St. Mary's Hospital's Catholic nuns in getting more medical care for black patients. Summing up his discussion, he talked candidly about how Palm Beach County always took care of it own.

There were no glory day stories and no name dropping of any kind. Dr. Brumback spoke gently and kindly about everyone. Along the way of his public health journey, he encountered a few set-backs, but only for a brief time, because he had an articulate and magical way of mediating. He would find the good in everyone and everything. The lecture lasted a couple of hours, but I could have listened to him discuss his vision for days. He gave me back the enthusiasm I had when I entered medical school. I came out of that lecture ready to work not for myself, but for my community. I was hooked to a public health career for life.

He was a man of intellect, a man of adventure and vision, a man of peace and mediation. When President Nixon asked Dr. Brumback to serve as the Public Health Doctor for the United States, he humbly declined saying he had much work to do in Palm Beach County. For him, it was not personal glory or compensation he sought, but rather he measured success in what the Health Department could do for the people. He was, in every sense of the word, a true public servant.

For those who knew Dr. Brumback knew he was a friend. He was approachable and willing to speak with anyone at any time. He knew how to listen and understand exactly what you needed. Dr. Brumback was able to balance work, family, church and his friends.

He often invited many of us to come dine at his new home at the Devonshire Living Facility at PGA National. On my last visit, we discussed a local radio interview I had made that very morning at 7:00 a.m. I told him I was astonished that he would have been up so early and even more astonished that he caught that particular radio interview. His comment to me was, "I have plenty of time on my hands to pay attention to these things now. I am glad I heard you speak. You did a really good job." Can you think of any kinder words? He was such a gentle and smart man.

Just like the Presidential Pen that President Lyndon Johnson used to sign the Migrant Health Act, which is mounted on the wall in the C.L. Brumback Health Center in Belle Glade, so will his legacy live on in each resident that comes through the Palm Beach County Residency Program.

We will miss you, dear friend and mentor.

Doctor Alina M. Alonso has been the Director of the Palm Beach County Health Department since 1989. She graduated from Barry University in 1978 with a Bachelor's of Science Degree in Biology. She received her medical degree in 1984 from the Universidad Autonoma de Cuidad Juarez in Mexico. She is a member of the faculty at Nova Southeastern University and Florida Atlantic University.

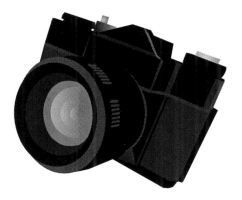

A Remembrance

By Richard Morgan, M.D.

April 26, 2011

Dear Editor-in-Chief,

As an eighty year-old reader of your excellent publication, I just wanted to send you a note to let you know I received your Healthy Stories books. I really appreciate you sending them to me.

I already recognize at least two of the stories (The Rat Lady and Rocky Raccoon), but I don't remember about the mouse escaping in the judge's chambers. I liked the Women, Infants and Children's story Triplets on a Plane, which reminded me that I started the first WIC program in Florida. At that time in the early 1970's, if I remember correctly, the USA Department of Agriculture started the program as a reimbursement program, which none of the health departments in Florida wanted to have anything to do with it, out of concerns of not being adequately and "timely" reimbursed, or did not have the monies up front to implement it. However, I convinced Dr. Milton Saslaw (Miami-Dade County Health Director and I was the Deputy County Health Director at that time) that the program was "badly" needed and he agreed we could start.

Other ideas for stories, you may recall, our efforts with the "Cuban boat list" back in 1980 (Mariel boatlift, I think), when as fast as FEMA opened up refugee shelters around Miami, we had to "shut" them down as they became very quickly "hell holes" of filth due to lack of adequate sanitary facilities, especially at the now demolished Orange Bowl, much was written about it in the Miami Herald at the time, the "measles report" I wrote for the Miami Grand Jury due to a complaint of a former health department employee, the lawyer for the grand jury was "amazed" by my report which squashed that complaint immediately.

The cancellation of our Robert Wood Johnson application for establishing "health clinics" in the public schools, which was to be an example for the foundation for use at other health departments to follow, but HRS Secretary Gregory Coler thought that the new Governor Martinez would find it unacceptable due to STD prevention and birth control counseling which might include the use of condoms and birth control pills, even though we had met with the school parents and included them in the planning and arranged for the requirement for signed and notarized permission for the students to participate in the clinics.

I can think of other possible stories such as, when I was the health department's representative for the monthly evening meetings of the Community Health Center of South Dade. There were about 15-20 people on the Health Center Board which represented various segments of the community and a number of them were "chain smokers", so that very quickly filled the board room with a haze of smoke. After several months of this, I proposed a "motion" that there would be no smoking during our meetings. I said, since we were a "health organization" concerned about the community's health, we should set the example for "healthy habits" at our monthly board meetings. After much deliberation my motion passed by a narrow majority and after the meeting I was accosted outside by at least two of the members who said that I was violating their "civil rights" to have the "pleasure of smoking" while participating in the meetings. I felt that they were verbally threatening me and I felt alarmed that the confrontation may escalate, therefore I quickly retreated back in to the board room where several of the members were still present and I waited until those two persons had left before getting into my car to return to my home in Miami Lakes. There were several attempts by these two people at subsequent meetings to "reconsider" the no-smoking policy" at the board meetings, but the majority of the members voted against reconsideration and I no longer felt threatened. Eventually, both of those two people resigned from the Board and we continued to have a smoke free environment at our Board meetings, including committee meetings. Also, at least for the subsequent years I served on the Board until I was appointed the Director of the Miami-Dade County Department of Public Health in 1976 and I appointed a replacement for me on the Board.

Another possible story comes to mind, Mort, if you recall, the health department was sued by the Miami Herald to require me to allow the newspaper representative to view the death certificate of a local surgeon who had died recently and it was rumored that he may have died of AIDS and possibly exposed his surgical patients to AIDS. I remember I was called to testify before the judge and you asked me if I "wore two hats", one as Health Department Director and one as Custodian of Vital Records for the county, which I did. The Miami Herald was claiming that they had a right to view the death record since the vital records law only said that a copy of the record could be provided to only persons who had a need to know, or something to that effect but no mention that anyone could not "see" the record. The local judge ruled in favor of the Miami Herald but the issue was appealed by the doctor's family and if I remember correctly it was finally settled by the Florida Supreme Court which ruled that the Miami Herald didn't have the right to even view the death certificate. You might check the records of the case; it could be a good story on how the department protected the confidentiality of vital records against the intrusion of "snooping" newspaper reporters.

Again, many thanks for the books which brought back many enjoyable memories.

Sincerely yours,

Richard Morgan, M.D.

Dr. Richard Morgan attended Emory University in Atlanta, Georgia where he received his undergraduate degree. In 1956 he graduated from Tulane University School of Medicine, New Orleans, Louisiana. He married Phyllis Ann Pittman of New Orleans, Louisiana in 1956 [soon to be wed 55 years this June 2011] and subsequently had three children, Mark, Scott, and Susan and seven grandchildren. Following medical school, he joined the US Army Medical Corp in June 1956. Dr. Morgan began Residency training in Military Preventive Medicine, which included obtaining a Master of Public Health degree from Tulane University School of Medicine in 1963. He retired from the US Army in 1968, with the rank of Lieutenant Colonel. Following army retirement he began as Assistant Director of The Dade County Department of Public Health in February 1970. In 1976, he was promoted the Director and served as Director until October 1987. He was appointed Clinical Associate and Clinical Professor, Department Of Epidemiology and Public Health, University of Miami School Of Medicine, 1974-1987. Dr. Morgan completed his public health career, 1988-1999, in Tampa, Florida, as a Senior Public Health Physician, serving in various capacities at The Hillsborough County Health Department, Tampa, Florida, and retired from the State of Florida in 1999. Since retirement he has participated in various community organizations in Tampa, including The New Tampa Rotary Club and as a board Member of The Tampa Chapter of The Military Officers Association of America.

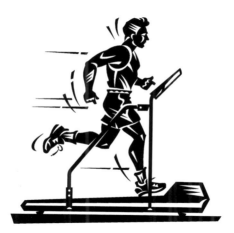

Let's Get Physical!

By Mort Laitner

I climb on the machine's deck, mounting it with all the determination of an Olympian, knowing for the next forty minutes the two of us will be one. Craning my neck downward, my index finger presses the large green square reading: "START." My fingers grasp the rails feeling the cold steel bars.

The machine's motor and belts groan and my legs commence walking. We merge at this leisurely pace while I ponder—quick weight loss program—four months—TWENTY POUNDS. Twenty pounds divided into $600 equals $30 dollars per pound. Well worth the money. I'd pay another $600 in a second to lose another twenty.

I wear my new forest green "Life is good" T-shirt, the one with Jake's picture on it. He's the stick figure with the infectious smile, now pedaling on a stationary bike on my shirt. I inhale the scent of the clean cotton. The shirt smells as fresh as if it were hung on an outdoor clothesline. The dry cotton cloth clings to my smaller body. I think, "life is good but it could be better. I've got to get off of this plateau."

Pushing the up arrow I increase the speed to two and a half miles per hour. My steps quicken as my body sends a message to my brain, "Great job, Mr. Fitness. In a few months you dropped more pounds than a bowling ball. Your heart loves it. Now it is time to hear some music."

My Blackberry rests on the treadmill console. I tap on it and Pandora appears. Beatles music fills my ears, replacing the monotonous hum of the treadmill. As I focus on the picture of the runner on the wall, memories of recent compliments bombard my brain.

"Wow! You look great!"
"How much weight have you lost?"
"What diet are you on?"
"Your face looks so much thinner."
"Your clothes are looking baggy."
"Better buy some new ones or go to the tailor."
"Now you are wearing a belt instead of those suspenders."

I start my reply with a simple, "Thanks, I'm trying to drop another twenty and it's tough right now because I've reached a plateau."

My index finger repeatedly presses the up. I hear the beep, beep, beep after every incremental increase, "As the machine's speed lands on 3.2 miles per hour. My legs quicken their pace as my heart starts rapid palpitations. My hungry lungs suck in deep breaths of fan generated air that crawls through my nose and flows out of my mouth.

After twenty minutes, my body heats up, my muscles tense, and my feet and knees begin to ache.

The Blackberry belts out:

"Let's get physical, physical.
I wanna get into physical.
Let me hear your body talk, body talk."

Droplets of perspiration bead on my forehead. They head toward my eyes as I picture Olivia Newton-John on MTV sweating in the gym surrounded by fat men. She wears a sexy smile, a tight blue and white exercise outfit and her signature headband. I recall her humorous aerobic anthem. The song won her a Grammy.

I remember dancing to Physical and seeing women wearing terry cloth headbands, trying to emulate Olivia's fashion statement. Hard to believe that was 1981.

I am not wearing a headband and sweat rolls into my eyes causing painful stings. My hand brushes against my eyes, throwing the sweat to the ground. Even Jake is soaked.

My thoughts turn to the cost of my treadmill, I realize what I had read is true. "[A]ging boomers . . . are willing to spend their resources to prevent the onset of chronic disease or lessen its severity if it already exists."*

I glance at the display, The digits blink—30 minutes—1.1 miles—201 calories. I think to myself, "Only another ten minutes to go on this maddening contraption." I remember reading about the history of treadmills, which were invented in the early 1800's to reform prisoners. I wonder about their success rate and laugh thinking about my attempts at physical reformation.

I continue jogging, pretending to be an astronaut living in the space station. NASA requires the astronauts to run on the treadmill as a counter measure against weightlessness. NASA even named their machine the Combined Operational Load Bearing External Resistance Treadmill (COLBERT). Should I follow NASA's lead and name my machine? I immediately think of calling it Olivia.

Droplets of human dew fall from my face and land on my gut. My body reeks of BO but I, like the Battery Bunny, just keep on going.

The odor triggers a synapse—my dilemma. I'm stuck on glacial-sized plateau called the 19, 20, 19, 20 plateau. My body weight is running in place. How do I climb to the 21 pound level?

As I contemplate my problem, the display blinks—42 minutes—279 calories—1.4 miles.

My time is up. I commence tapping on the down arrow until the motor yawns. Now the beeps are music to my ears. I hit the red stop button, dismount and head for the pool. After swimming a few laps, my body cools. I dry off and head to the couch where I sit feeling the exhilaration of good health.

No longer contemplating my dilemma, I realize I have not felt this good in decades.

My body has spoken. Life is good. ☀

* Morrison, Eileen E., Ethics in Health Administration A Practical Approach Decision Makers, Jones & Bartlett Publishers, (2006) p. 113.

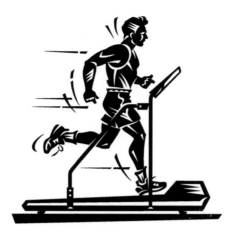

¡Vayamos a lo Físico!

Por Mort Laitner
Traducido por Ninfa Urdaneta

Yo me monto en la plataforma de la máquina, haciéndolo con toda la determinación de un jugador olímpico, sabiendo que por los próximos cuarenta y cinco minutos los dos de nosotros seremos uno. Inclinando mi cuello hacia abajo, mi dedo índice presiona el cuadrado verde grande que dice: "INICIO." Mis dedos agarran los rieles sintiendo las frías barras de acero.

El motor de la máquina y las correas comenzaron a resonar y mis piernas comenzaron a caminar. Nos fusionamos sin prisas, mientras yo considero---programa de rápida perdida de peso---cuatro meses---VEINTE LIBRAS. Veinte libras divididas entre $600 son $30 dólares por libra. Vale la pena por esta cantidad de dinero. Yo pagaría otros $600 en un segundo a fin de perder otras veinte.

Yo uso mi camiseta de color verde que dice "La Vida es Buena," la que tiene el retrato de Jake en ella. El es el de la figura y sonrisa pegajosa, ahora pedaleando en una bicicleta estática sobre mi camiseta. Yo inhalo la esencia del limpio algodón. La camisa huele tan fresca como si estuviera colgada en un cordón de ropa a la intemperie. Yo pienso, "la vida es buena pero puede ser mejor. Me tengo que deshacer de este estancamiento."

Presionando la flecha hacia arriba yo incremento la velocidad a dos y media millas por hora. Mis pasos se hacen más rápidos mientras mi cuerpo le envía un mensaje a mi cerebro, "Buen trabajo Sr. De Buen Estado Físico. En unos meses has bajado más libras que una bola de Bowling. Tu corazón lo agradece. Ahora es hora de oír un poco de música."

Mi Blackberry está en la consola de la trotadora. Yo lo toco y aparece Pandora. La música de los Beatles llena mis oídos, remplazando el monótono zumbido de la trotadora. Mientras me enfoco en la foto sobre la pared, las memorias de recientes complementos bombardean mi cerebro.

"¡Wow! ¡Te ves muy bien!"
"¿Cuánto peso has perdido?"
"¿Qué dieta estás haciendo?"
"Tu cara se ve mucho más delgada."
"Tus ropas se ven bastante holgadas."
"Mejor que compres unas nuevas o vayas al sastre."
"Ahora estás usando un cinturón en lugar de esos tirantes suspendedores."

Yo comienzo mi respuesta con un simple, "Gracias. Estoy tratando de bajar otras veinte y es difícil ahora porque me he estancado."

Mi dedo índice repetidamente presiona el botón hacia arriba. Yo oigo el beep, beep, beep después de cada incremento gradual. Mientras la velocidad de la máquina alcanza 3.2 millas por hora. Mis piernas apuran el paso mientras mi corazón empieza a palpitar rápidamente. Mis pulmones hambrientos respiran profundamente chupando aire generado por ventilador que entra lentamente a través de mi nariz y sale por mi boca.

Después de veinte minutos mi cuerpo se acalora, mis músculos se tensan, y mis pies y rodillas me comienzan a doler.

El Blackberry canta a grito pelado:

"Let's get physical, physical.
I wanna get into physical.
Let me hear your body talk, body talk."

Gotas de transpiración de sudor en mi frente. Ellas se dirigen hacia mis ojos mientras me imagino un retrato de Olivia Newton-John en MTV sudando en el gimnasio rodeada de hombres gordos. Ella tiene una sonrisa sexy, ropa ajustada para hacer ejercicio de color azul y blanca y su típica bandana en su frente. Recuerdo su himno aeróbico de gran humor. Ella ganó un Grammy por esta canción.

Recuerdo bailar Physical y ver mujeres usando bandanas de tela de toalla, tratando de seguir la moda impuesta por Olivia. Difícil de creer que eso era en 1981.

No estoy usando una bandana y el sudor va hacia adentro de mis ojos causando doloroso ardor. Mis manos limpian mis ojos, tirando el sudor al suelo. Inclusive Jake está empapado.

Mis pensamientos se van hacia el costo de la trotadora, Me doy cuanta lo que había leído recientemente en el periódico, que la generación de la post guerra que se avejenta ... está dispuesta a gastar sus recursos a fin de evitar el surgimiento de enfermedades crónicas o disminuir su severidad si ya ellas existen.

Yo doy una mirada a la pantalla los dígitos titilan—30 minutes—1.1 millas—201 calorías. Yo pienso, "Solo diez minutos más en este exasperante aparato." Yo recuerdo leer acerca de la historia de las trotadoras, las cuales fueron inventadas a principios de lo 1,800's para reformar prisioneros. Me pregunto acerca de su éxito y me río acerca de los intentos de reformarme físicamente.

Yo continúo trotando pretendiendo ser un astronauta viviendo en una estación espacial. La NASA requiere a los astronautas correr en una trotadora como medida contra la ingravidez. La NASA llamó a su máquina la Combined Operational Load Bearing External Resistance Treadmill (COLBERT). ¿Debería yo seguir los pasos de la NASA y ponerle un nombre a mi máquina? Yo inmediatamente pienso en llamarla Olivia.

Gotas de rocío humano caen de mi cara y aterrizan en mi barriga. Mi cuerpo apesta a hedor corporal pero yo, como la Battery Bunny, sigo andando.

El olor genera una transmisión neural—mi dilema. Estoy atascado en una meseta glacial llamada el estancamiento de 19, 20, 19, 20. Mi peso corporal está corriendo en el mismo lugar. ¿Cómo hago para alcanzar la libra del nivel 21?

Mientras contemple mi problema, la pantalla titila—42 minutes—279 calorías—1.4 miles.

Mi sesión terminó. Yo comienzo a tocar la flecha que disminuye la velocidad hasta que el motor se apaga. Ahora los beeps son música para mis oídos. Yo presiono el botón rojo de pare, me bajo y me dirijo a la piscina. Después de nadar varias vueltas mi cuerpo se enfría. Me seco y me dirijo al sofá en el cual me siento sintiendo la vibración de la buena salud.

Ya no contemplando mi dilema, me doy cuenta que no he sentido este bien en décadas.

Mi cuerpo ha hablado. La vida es buena.

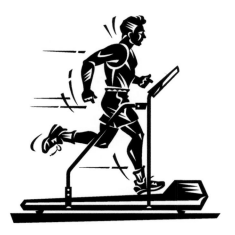

An Nou Bay Kò Nou Mouvman Egzèsis!

Se Mort Laitner ki ekri istwa sa a
Translation Roland Pierre

Mwen monte sou plato machin pou fè egzèsis la mwen monte sou machin la ak konviksyon yon mon ki ap patisipe nan jwèt olenpik yo. Paske mwen konen ke pou karant minit ki ap vini yo mwen menm ak machin egzèsisi la pral fè yon sèl. Lè mwen panche tèt mwen anba, dwèt endèx mwen peze bouton kare ki koulè vèt la epi ki make" KOMANSE". Dwèt mwen kenbe balistrad machin pou fè egzèsis la lè sa a mwen santi fè balistrad la ki frèt anba men mwen.

Motè machin la ak sentiron machin la gronde epi tou janb mwen komanse ap mache. Nou ap kontinye ti pa ti pa nan kadans mwen te pran an pandan ke mwen te ap reflechi ---pwogram pou moun pèdi pwa vit—kat mwa—VEN LIV—Ven liv divize pa 600 dola egal 30 dola pou ckal liv. Sa byen vo lajan sa a. Mwen tap menm peye yon lòt 600 dola nan yon segond pou mwen te kapab pèdi yon lòt ven liv.

Mwen abiye ak mayo vèt koulè fèy bwa ki make sou li "La vi a bèl" sa menm ki gen foto Jak sou li a. Sou mayo ki sou mwen a Jak se yon figi tankou yon bout bwa ak yon souri ki atrapan sou li ki ap pedale bisiklèt ki ret anplas yo.

Mwen rale lè pou mwen byen respire sant koton pwòp mayo a. Mayo a santi bon tankou si yo te tann li sou liyn nan lakou pou li seche. Twal koton mayo a kole sou kò mwen ki vinn pi piti a. Mwen di tèt mwen ke "lavi a bèl men ke li ta kab pi bèl toujou. Mwen dwe soti sou plato machin pou fè egzèsis la"

Lè sa a mwen peze flèch ki ap gade anwo a mwen ogmante vitès la a de mil e demi pa è de tan. Pye mwen yo ap prale pi vit pandan ke kò mwen ap voye yon mesaj bay sèvo mwen, «bon travay Mesye anfòm. Nan kèk mwa ou pèdi plis pwa ke yon boul moun sèvi pou jwe jwèt boling la.Kè ou renmen sa anpil.Kounye a se lè pou ou tande enpe mizik"

Telefon blakberi mwen a rete sou etajè machin pou fè egzèsis la. Men apiye sou li epi Pandora parèt Mizik mizisyen Beatles ranpli zorèy mwen epi li ranplase grondman ke machin pou fè egzèsis la te ap fè. Pandan ke mwen ap konsantre, lide mwen sou foto moun ki ap kouri ki sou mi a souvni tout konpliman ke mwen te resevwa ap bonbade sèvo mwen.

"Wow! Ou parèt anfòm!"
"Ki kantite pwa ke ou pèdi?"
"Kilès dayèt ke ou ap fè?"
"Figi ou parèt pi mens."
"Rad sou ou parèt two gran pou ou."
"Pitou ou al achte lòt rad ou byen al fè fèmen yo."
"Kounye a ou mete yon sentiron angiz bretèl yo."

Mwen te toujou reponn «Mèsi mwen ap eseye pèdi yon lòt ven liv epi li difisil anpil paske mwen rive nan bout mwen"

Dwèt endèx mwen an plizyè fwa peze bouton pou fè machin la al pi vit la. Mwen tande bip, bip, bip chak fwa ke vitès la ogmante. Pandan ke machin la ap monte vitès li sou 3.2 mil pa è de tan. Janb mwen yo al pi vit pandan ke kè mwen komanse palpitasyon rapid. Poumon mwen yo ki swaf lè ap ranmase lè a ap rale lè a jouk nan fon apre ke li finn pase nan nen mwen epi sòti nan bouch mwen.

Apre trant minit, kò mwen chofe, miskl mwen yo gen kranp, mwen gen doulè nan pye mwen ak jenou mwen.

Telefòn blakbery a ap bay mizik :

"An nou bay kò nou mouvman.
Mwen pral bay kò mwen mouvman
Kite mwen tande kò ou ki ap pale"

Gout syè mouye figi mwen. Yo ap koule nan je mwen pandan ke mwen ap fè vizyon Olivia Newton-John nan estasyon television MTV ki ap sye nan gym la kote ke li antoure ak gason ki twò gwo. Li gen sou figi li yon souri ki trè sexy epi li mete sou li yon rad ble ak blan ki sere sou kò li pou fè egzèsis epi li gen nan tèt li yon bando ke li menm sèlman genyen. Mwen sonje chante pou moun fè egzèsis ke li te konn chante a e ki te lakòz ke li te genyen yon pri pou chantè ke yo rele Grammy.

Mwen sonje ke mwen te konn danse chante ki te rele Physical la epi ke mwen te konn wè fanm yo ki te gen nan tèt yo bando ki fèt ak twal sèvyèt ki te tankou sa Olivia Newton-John te konn mete a, li difisil pou mwen kwè ke se te ane 1981.

Mwen pa gen yon bando nan tèt mwen pou anpeche syè a koule sou je mwen, epi lè syè a koule nan je mwen li pike je mwen anpil. Mwen siye ak men mwen syè ki sou je mwen a epi mwen voye syè a tonbe atè. Menm foto Jak ki sou mayo a mouye ak syè.

Lide mwen al tounen sou sa machin pou fè egzèsis la koute mwen, mwen realize ke sa mwen te li a se vre "Moun ki ap gran moun ki te fèt nan lane yo rele boomers yo...pa gen pwoblèm pou yo depanse lajan yo pou evite ke maladi kronik antre sou yo oswa pou anpeche ke li vinn pi grav si ke maladi a déjà egziste sou yo "*

Mwen gade ekran machin pou fè egzèsis la chif yo tenyen—trant minit—1.1mil—201 calories. Mwen di tèt mwen , "Sèlman dis minit ankò pou mwen rete sou machin egzèsis sa a." Mwen sonje ke mwen te li istwa machin pou fè egzèsis yo rele treadmills, ke yo te envante nan ane 1800's yo pou refòme prizonye. Mwen mande tèt mwen eske yo te reisi fè prizonye yo refòme ak machin sa yo lè ke mwen te sonje jan ke mwen te eseye refòme kò mwen pou li fè egzèsis.

Mwen kontinye ap kouri sou machin pou fè egzèsis la mwen ap fè tèt mwen kwè ke mwen se te yon astronòt ki te ap viv nan estasyon nan lespas. Òganizasyon ki okipe bagay nan lespas ke yo rele NASA egzije ke astronòt kouri sou yon machin treadmill pou yo kontrarye zefè ke moun nan pa gen pwa ditou lè ke li nan lespas. NASA te menm rele machin yo a Combined Operational Load Bearing External Resistance Treadmill (COLBERT). Eske se pou mwen te fè tankou NASA te fè epi rele machin mwen a yon non? Menm moman a mwen di tèt mwen ke mwen ta rele li Olivia.

Gout syè tonbe sou figi mwen epi yo ateri sou lestomak mwen. Kò mwen santi fò ak odè syè men tankou ti lapen ki mache ak batri a mwen kontinye fè sa ke mwen te ap fè a.

Odè syè voye yon siyal bay sèvo mwen--- dilèm pa mwen a. Mwen kole sou you plato ki gwose yo mòn glas se yon plato ki rele 19,20, 19, 20 plato. Pwa mwen ap kanpe an plas li pa chanje di tou. Kijan pou mwen monte nan wotè 21 liv la?

Pandan ke mwen ap kontanple dilèm mwen a ekran a tenyen —42 minit—279 kalori—1.4 mil.

Lè pou mwen fini a te rive. Mwen komanse apiye sou bouton pou bese vitès la jouktan motè a baye. Kounye a bwi bip yo se yon misik pou zorèy mwen. Mwen peze bouton rouj pou fè machin la rete, desan machin pou egzèsis la epi mwen pran wout pou mwen ale nan pisin la. Apre ke mwen naje kèk bras kò mwen refwadi. Mwen seche kò mwen epi mwen al chita sou sofa a pandan ke mwen santi ke yon sansasyon bon lasante anvahi kò mwen.

Paske mwen pate genyen yon dilèm pou trakase mwen, mwen te realize ke gen lontan plis ke dizan depi ke mwen te santi mwen byen konsa.

Kò mwen te pale. Lavi a bèl. ☼

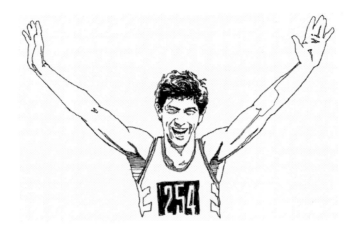

Ben's Story

By Neal Greene

For years I've been watching my youngest (of three) sons compete in sports: BMX bike racing, skiing, baseball, basketball, soccer, football and all the backyard hopping and skipping around to climbing trees. Ben always finished dead last. During most of these competitions Ben cried furiously out of frustration because his damaged body would not allow him to actually compete to win. Junior high school was probably the worst time for Ben because the kids at that age were downright mean. Mocking and laughing made him more self-conscious than he already was.

Ben was born three months premature because his mom died of a brain aneurysm at the dinner table. She had zero brain activity by the time the ambulance got her to the hospital. Doctors worked vigorously for a short time, knowing this woman, wife, daughter, and mother was not going to live much longer.

One of the doctors came to me and said, "Your wife is not going to make it. Would you like us to try and save the baby?" What a question. At that moment, I couldn't even see straight from the shock, horror, and stress of what had just happened. I was so confused, but I agreed.

Ben was removed by Caesarean section and rushed to a neo-natal clinic one-hundred miles away. I stayed at home trying to keep my sanity while comforting my four and five year-olds. Each night, always at dinner time, the phone rang and nurses or doctors plead with me to visit Ben, who at that time, they thought probably would not make it. Most preemies of that status live only to have cerebral palsy, deafness, blindness, or retardation. Many just die.

The year before my wife passed away, we lost a son that was born full term and died of unknown causes in the hospital, hours after birth. The new baby's room was fully decorated with clothes in his closet and much happy anticipation of his arrival in the house. Explaining that to my sons was hell. Now, here we were again, but without Mom, and I was supposed to get excited over this new baby? "I don't think so."

Night after night, the calls came from the hospital and staff pleaded, "Please come and bond with your son."

"Is he going to live?" I'd ask.

"We don't know yet," they replied. Not good enough. I stayed home with my boys.

Shortly after Ben's arrival at the neo-natal clinic, the phone calls changed. Now the doctors wanted my permission to give Ben an experimental drug that could save his life. An extract from sheep, injected into Ben, would somehow speed up the development of his lungs. Finally, out of sheer exhaustion, I agreed. Within twenty-four hours, the doctors were pleased with Ben's development. Absolutely amazing! After about a week, the phone calls started again to encourage us to come and visit. His prognosis was still iffy, to say the least. The doctors felt he would survive, but were unsure what his quality of life would be.

One afternoon, I told his two brothers that we were going to visit Ben. Once at the hospital, I mustered up my strength and smilingly walked into the room where Ben was.

"Oh my God!"

His flesh was so thin I could see his organs. Flesh? It was just a thin layer of skin. He had no flesh. I reached down with one finger and very gently stroked his arm. Immediately, monitors started screeching throughout the room. My boys and I freaked out. Nurses came rushing in and told us we couldn't stimulate him.

"How are we supposed to 'bond' with him if we can't touch him?" I asked.

"Just being here is enough," we were told. "He knows you're here."

Ben was released from the neo-natal clinic almost three months later and was sent to our local hospital for another month where nurses referred to him as the Miracle Baby. Doctors said Ben had mild cerebral palsy. They would know what parts of his body would be affected the worst.

"If he can keep up with his peers, then he will be fine," they said.

His cerebral palsy made it rough for Ben, but he always prevailed. Working twice as hard, he succeeded. In the final analysis, Ben's weakness was in his legs, hips and ankles. He would trip when walking up stairs and ran like a three-legged goat.

In November of 2008, Ben announced to his friends, family, and the world, "I am competing in an IRONMAN event in Tempe, Arizona."

He trained relentlessly for that year. Triathlons, marathons, whatever he could do to strengthen himself. As a full time student at Arizona State University, Ben majored in Health and Wellness. He wanted to help kids with similar challenges. He also worked full time and bought his own equipment: bikes, wetsuits, helmets, the works.

Sixteen hours and eleven minutes into the race, Ben collapsed over the finish line. He became a 2009 FORD IRONMAN FINISHER!

Ben continues his training and schooling while raising money for ENDURE TO CURE (pediatric cancer).

Ben has been told by so many supporting team and sport members to tell his story, but Ben remains low key. Well, I'm his father, and I felt that his story needed to be told.

"Ben, you are an inspiration to many and my hero. Bravo, my son." ✨

Neal Greene is an artist who lives in Peoria, Arizona. His artwork hangs in the White House. He has re-married and is now the proud father of four. His website is www.outofmygourdcreations.com.

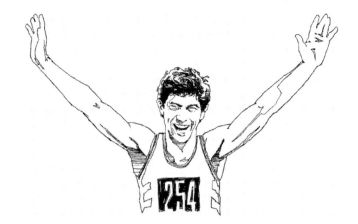

La Historia de Ben

Por Neal Greene
Traducido por Frank Menendez y Francisco Menendez

Durante años he estado viendo a mi hijo, el más pequeño de tres, compitiendo en deportes: carreras de bicicletas BMX, esquí, béisbol, baloncesto, fútbol, fútbol americano así como los saltos y las trepadas de árboles. Ben siempre terminó en último lugar. Durante la mayor parte de estas competiciones Ben gritaba con furia de frustración porque su cuerpo dañado no le permitía competir realmente para ganar. La escuela secundaria fue probablemente el peor momento para Ben, porque los niños a esa edad eran francamente malos. La burla y la risa lo hizo más consciente de lo que Ben ya era.

Ben nació prematuramente, con tres meses, porque su madre murió de un aneurisma cerebral cuando estaba cenando en casa. Ella tenía cero actividad cerebral en el momento en que la ambulancia la llevó al hospital. Los médicos trabajaron enérgicamente para salvarla, a sabiendas de que esta mujer, esposa, hija y madre no iba a vivir por mucho más.

Uno de los médicos se me acercó y me dijo: "Tu esposa no va a sobrevivir. ¿Le gustaría que trate de salvar al bebé? "¡Qué pregunta! En ese momento, yo ni siquiera podía ver correctamente por el shock, el horror, y el estrés por lo que había sucedido. Yo estaba tan confundido, pero estuve de acuerdo.

Ben fue retirado por cesárea y se lo llevaron a una clínica neonatal cien millas de distancia. Me quedé en casa tratando de mantener mi cordura mientras reconfortaba a mis hijos de cuatro y cinco años de edad. Cada noche, siempre a la hora de cenar, sonó el teléfono y las enfermeras o los médicos me rogaban que visitara a Ben, que en ese momento, pensaban que probablemente no sobreviviría. La mayoría de los bebés prematuros que viven tienen parálisis cerebral, sordera, ceguera o retraso mental. Muchos acaban en la muerte.

Tres año antes de que mi esposa murió, perdimos a un hijo que nació a término y murió por causas desconocidas en el hospital, horas después del nacimiento. La habitación del recién nacido estaba decorada por completo, con la ropa en su armario y eramos muy felices anticipando su llegada a casa. Explicarle eso a mis hijos fue un infierno. Ahora, aquí estamos otra vez, pero sin madre, y se suponía que estuviera emocionado por este nuevo bebé? "Yo no lo creo."

Noche tras noche, las llamadas provenían del hospital y el personal me decía: "Por favor, venga y déle compañía a su hijo."

"¿Es que va a vivir?" Les preguntaba.

"No sabemos todavía", respondieron. Pero como aquello no era suficiente para mí, me quedé en casa con mis hijos.

Poco después de la llegada de Ben a la clínica neonatal, las llamadas telefónicas cambiaron. Ahora los médicos querían mi permiso para darle a Ben una droga experimental que podría salvar su vida. Un extracto de oveja se inyecta en Ben, y de alguna manera eso aceleraría el desarrollo de sus pulmones. Finalmente, por puro agotamiento, acepté. Dentro de las veinticuatro horas, los médicos estaban satisfechos con el desarrollo de Ben. ¡Absolutamente increíble! Después de una semana, las llamadas telefónicas comenzaron de nuevo animándonos a que lo visitáramos. Su pronóstico era dudoso todavía, por decir lo menos. Ahora los médicos creían que iba a sobrevivir, pero no estaban seguros de las limitaciones que Ben tendría.

Una tarde, les dije a sus dos hermanos que iban a visitar a Ben. Una vez en el hospital, reuní mis fuerzas y con una sonrisa entre en la habitación donde estaba Ben.

"!Oh, Dios mío!"

Su piel era tan fina que podía ver sus órganos. Él no tenía carne. Me agaché con un dedo y suavemente le acaricié el brazo. Inmediatamente, los monitores comenzaron a sonar por toda la habitación. Mis hijos y yo nos asustamos. Las enfermeras llegaron corriendo y nos dijeron que no podíamos tocarlo.

"¿Cómo se supone que pueda haber vínculo afectivo con él si no lo puedo tocar?" Pregunté.

"Sólo estar aquí es suficiente", nos dijeron. "Él sabe que están aquí."

Ben salió de la clínica neonatal casi tres meses después y fue enviado a nuestro hospital durante un mes donde las enfermeras se referían a él como el bebé milagro. Los médicos dijeron que Ben tenía un nivel leve de parálisis cerebral. Ellos sabrían qué parte de su cuerpo seria la pero afectada.

"Si es capaz de mantenerse al mismo nivel de sus compañeros, entonces va a estar bien", dijeron.

Su parálisis cerebral era difícil para Ben, pero siempre prevaleció. Trabajando el doble, lo lograba. En el análisis final, la debilidad de Ben estaba en sus piernas, caderas y tobillos. Él tropezaba al subir escaleras y corría como una cabra con tres patas.

En noviembre de 2008, Ben anunció a sus amigos, familia, y al el mundo: "Estoy compitiendo en un evento Ironman, en Tempe, Arizona."

Entrenó sin descanso durante ese año. Triatlones, maratones, todo lo que podía hacer para fortalecerse. Como estudiante en la Universidad Estatal de Arizona, Ben se especializó en salud y bienestar. Quería ayudar a los niños con problemas similares. También trabajaba para comprarse su propio equipo: bicicletas, trajes de neopreno, casco, de todo.

A las dieciséis horas y once minutos de la carrera, Ben se desplomó sobre la línea de meta. ¡Se convirtió en un ACABADOR DEL 2009 FORD IRONMAN!

Ben continúa su formación y educación, mientras que recauda dinero para la fundación ENDURE TO CURE (cáncer pediátrico).

Ben ha sido contactado por varios miembros de soporte y miembros de deportes para que cuente su historia, pero Ben se mantiene censillo. Bueno, yo soy su padre, y sentí que esta historia tenia que contarse.

"Ben, eres una inspiración para muchos y mi héroe. Bravo, hijo mío."

Neal Greene es un artista que vive en Peoria, Arizona. Su obra cuelga en la Casa Blanca. Ha vuelto a casarse y es ahora el orgulloso padre de cuatro. Su página de web es www.outofmygourdcreations.com.

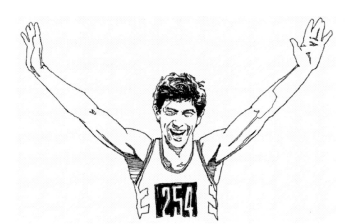

Istwa Ben

Se Neal Greene ki ekri istwa sa a
Translation Roland Pierre

Pandan plizyè ane mwen te ap gade pi jenn nan pitit gason mwen yo(mwen gen twa) al fè konpetisyon nan esp: kous bisiklèt BMX, ski, bezbòl, foutbòl, foutbòl ameriken epi sote nan lakou dèyè a epi vole pou li grenpe sou pye bwa. Ben te toujou fini andènye. Pandan laplipa konpetisyon yo Ben te toujou ap rele paske li te gen anpil fristrasyon avèk kò li ki te domaje e ki pa te pèmet li lite byen pou li genyen jwèt la. Pandan ke li te nan lekòl segondè se te pi move epòk pou li paske ti moun laj say o te san pitye epi yo te mechan. Lè ke yo te ap ri li, ap pase li nan betiz sa te fè ke li te plis rann li kont nan ki eta ke li te ye.

Ben te fèt twa mwa avan tèm paske manman li te mouri ak yon aneurism kidonk yon venn nan sèvo li ki te pete pandan ke li te ap manje a tab. Sèvo manman Ben li pa te gen okenn aktivite lè ke yo te mennen fanm ansent la lopital nan anbilans la. Doktè yo te travay anpil ak tout kouraj yo pandan yon ti ka dè paske yo te konnen ke fanm sa a,madanm la, pitit fi a, epi manman ke li te ye a pa tap viv lontan apre ke yo te mennen li lopital la.

Gen yonn nan doktè yo ki vinn jwenn mwen epi ki di mwen

"Madanm ou pap chape. Eske ou vle ke nou eseye sove ti bebe a?" Ki kalite keksyon sa a. Lè sa a mwen pa te kab wè klè akòz shòk, ledè, epi estrès ke sa ki te ap pase a te ban mwen. Mwen te egare san ke mwen pa konnen sa ke mwen te ap di men mwen di dakò sove ti moun nan.

Yo te fè yon sezaryèn pou retire Ben nan vant manman li epi yo te kouri ak li nan kote yo okipe ti moun ki pa tèm ak ki fèk fèt yo ke yo rele klinik neo-natal ki te tabli san mil de lopital la. Mwen te rete lakay mwen ap eseye kenbe tèt mwen pou li pa pati pandan ke mwen te ap konsole pitit mwen yo ki te gen kat ak senkan. Chak swa a lè ke nou te ap manje telefòn la te konn sonnen epi se te doktè ak enfimyè yo ki te konn ap rele pou yo laprye mwen pou mwen al vizite Ben ke yo kwè ki pa tap chape lè sa a. Laplipa timoun prematire ki te fèt tankou Ben te konn chape men yo te konn paralize nan sèvo yo, yo soud, avèg, oswa retade entatad. Anpil te konn mouri

Nan menm lane ke madanm mwen te mouri a nou te pèdi yon timoun ki te fèt tèm epi ki te mouri kèk è de tan apre ke li te fèt la pou yon rezon ke nou pa te konnen. Nou te byen dekore chanb pou ti bebe a epi te gen rad nan bifèt la pou ti bebe a epi tout moun te ap tann ti bebe a vini ak kè kontan. Lè sa a se te yon lanfè pou mwen te esplike lòt ti moun mwen yo ke ti bebe a te mouri. Kounye a pou nou rekòmanse ankò nan menm bagay sa a, epi an plis san ke manman yo pa te la. Eske mwen te sipoze gen kè kontan nan tann ti bebe sa kounye? "Mwen pa kwè sa a".

Nwit apre nwit lopital la tap rele yo te ap laprye mwen, "Tanpri vini epi fè ti moun nan abitye ak ou".

"Eske li ap viv ?" mwen te mande

"Nou pako konnen" yo te konn reponn mwen. Repons la pa te ase bon pou mwen. Mwen te rete lakay la ak lòt pitit gason mwen yo.

Kèk tan apre ke Ben te rive nan sèvis neonatal lopital la kout telefòn yo te chanje kounye a doktè yo te ap mande mwen pèmisyon pou yo bay Ben yon medikaman ke doktè te fèk ap eseye e ki te kab sove lavi li. Yon pwodwi ke yo retire nan mouton te kab devlope poumon li yo si yo te bay Ben yon piki ak li. Alafen mwen te tèlman bouke ak doktè yo ki te ap rele mwen ke mwen di ke mwen te dakò pou yo ba li medikaman yo te ap eseye a. Apre vennkatrè doktè yo te kontan pou jan ke Ben te ap devlope a. Vreman extraòdinè! Apre yon semenn, telefòn la sonnen ankò pou ankouraje nou pou al vizite

Ben. Yo pa te bay garanti ke li te ap sove. Doktè yo te kwè ke li te kapab sove men yo pa te konnen si li pa tap kokobe.

Yon apremidi mwen di de frè li yo ke nou ta pral rann Ben vizit lopital la. Yon fwa ke mwen te rive lopital la mwen ranmase kouraj mwen ak de men mwen epi ak yon souri sou bouch mwen mwen antre pou wè Ben.

"O Bondye!"

Po li te tèlman fen ke men te kab wè tout ògàn li yo kidonk pati kò li yo ki te andedan li a. Vyann? li se te yo kabwèt zo ak po. Mwen lonje yon dwèt mwen epi mwen teke bra li. Menm moman a tout aparèy ki te sou ti bebe a pou gade kijan kè li ak lòt pati nan kò, li te ap fonktyonnen te komanse ap fè bwi nan chanb lopital la. Laperèz te pran mwen menm ak pitit gason mwen yo. Enfimyè a vini li di ke nou pa te kab manyen ti bebe a.

"Kijan ke nou ap kab abitye ak ti bebe a si ke nou pa kapab manyen li?" mwen te mande.

"Sèlman vini wè li epi kanpe bòkote li se kont "yo te di nou" li konnen ke nou la"

Ben te pase twa mwa nan sèvis neonatal la epi apre sa yo te mete li nan yon lopital tou pre lakay la pandan yon mwa, kote sa a enfimyè yo te rele li Ti Bebe Mirakl la.Doktè yo di ke Ben te gen enpe sèvo li ki te paralize.Yo te kwèke se apre ke yo ta va konnen ki pati nan kò li ki te ap domaje plis.

Si li kapab fè sa ke lòt timoun laj li ak kondisyon li fè li ap san pwoblèm.

Sèvo li ki te paralyze te fè ke lavi a te di pou Ben men li te pote laviktwa.Li te travay de fwa pi di men li te krye viktwa. Apre ke Ben te soti lopital se te janb li, hanch li ak jwenti pye li ki te fèb e ki te ba li pwoblèm. Lè pou li te monte eskalye li te konn ap tonbe epi lè ke li te ap kouri li te tankou yon kabrit ki te genyen twa pye.

Nan mwa Novanb 2008, Ben te anonse zanmi li, ak fanmi, ak tout moun sou latè "Mwen prale nan konpetisyon yo rele IRON-MAN ki ap fèt nan Tempe nan Arizona".

Pandan ane a li antrene tèt li san pran souf. Li fè Triathlons, marathons, tout kalite espò li te kab fè pou li fòtifye kò li. Lè ke Ben se te yon etidyan ki ap etidye full time ki te ap pran anpil lè klas nan Arizona State University, Ben te ap etidye Lasante ak Byen-nèt. Li te vle ede lòt ti moun ki te gen menm pwoblem nan kò yo ke li te genyen a. Pandan ke li se te yon etidyan ki ap fè anpil lè lekòl li te ap travay anpil lè tou, full time, epi ak kòb travay li li te achte pwòp ekipman pa li: bisiklèt, rad pou moun fè espò, chapo an metal ki pwoteje tèt moun ak tout lòt kalite ekipman.

Sèzè de tan epi onz minit nan kous la Ben te tonbe sou liyn pou moun fini kous la li te vini yonn nan moun ki te fini kous la sa yo rele yon 2009 FORD IRONMAN FINISHER!

]Ben te kontinye ap antrene li epi ap etidye lekòl pandan ke li te ap fè aktivite pou ranmase lajan pou yon òganizasyon ki ede ti moun ki gen maladi kanè yo rele ENDURE TO CURE.

Anpil moun ki sipòte ekip li a ak lòt moun ki fè espò ak li te di Ben pou li rakonte istwa li a, men Ben pa vle fè twòp bwi ak sa. Ebyen mwen se papa li, epi mwen santi ke istwa li a merite pou ke yo rakonte li.

Ben ou se yon moun ki se yon modèl pou lòt moun ki enspire anpil moun epi ou se ewo mwen. Bravo pitit gason mwen. ☼

Neal Greene se yon atist ki abite nan Peoria, Arizona. Tablo li ak lòt èv li koke nan White House ki se palè nasyonal peyiAmeriken. Li remarye epi kounye a li se yon papa ki fyè de se ke li gen kat pitit.Adrès nan entènèt li sewww. outofmygourdcreations.com.

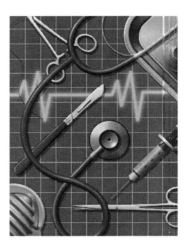

Not A Big Deal

By Faten Hamam

It was October 8, 2008, I was at my office in Jeddah, Saudi Arabia when I heard my cell phone rang nonstop. I asked my friend to answer it. My friend entered my office with a worried look on her face. She said, "It's your husband, Bandar. He says it's urgent."

I picked up the receiver and heard my husband's voice. His tone told me that there was something terribly wrong. In a trembling voice, he whispered, "Sara died today."

My heart fell to the floor. This was like a nightmare, and I wanted to wake up. I was speechless. My words refused to come out of my mouth. Finally, I just said, "I'll be home shortly."

As I hung up the phone I tried to remain calm. I was in shock. I couldn't believe Sara died. We were like sisters and in fact, she was my sister-in-law. She was the one who introduced me to my husband. We attended university together. My husband and I were traumatized by this tragedy.

Sara died from complications after delivering her baby. Her baby would never see her mother because of an error committed by a doctor.

Sara's tragedy started on October 2 at 2:15 AM when she woke experiencing something strange she never felt before. Sara woke her husband, Josef, and told him. Both were terrified as they thought something was wrong with her pregnancy. This was their first baby, and they were so happy and excited to become parents. He called 911 and explained, "My wife is 8 months pregnant and is in severe pain. Please come as fast as you can!"

Within fifteen minutes, an ambulance arrived and the paramedics said, "Sara is going to have her baby. We are taking her to the nearest hospital." Josef called Sara's mom, his parents and my husband to ask us all to meet at the hospital.

At 3:00 AM, a nurse came and rolled Sara to the delivery room to prepare her while Josef filled out the paperwork at the registration office. We all arrived shortly thereafter. Josef rushed to the delivery room to be with his wife. A couple of hours later, he entered the waiting room to inform us, "I just spoke to Dr. Jamal and he has decided that Sara isn't progressing fast enough, so she needs a cesarean section."

At 8:00 AM, Josef came out again and exclaimed, "Sara gave birth to a very beautiful girl. Sara is still unconscious from the operation."

At 10:30 AM, Sara and her baby were in their room when she finally woke surrounded by everyone who congratulated her. "Her name is Sereen," said Sara elatedly. Sara's mother started to give her some advice about how to raise her baby and what she should and shouldn't do.

On October 6, Dr. Jamal stopped by to check on Sara. She complained to him, "I'm still having very strong pain."

The physician replied, "Its nothing serious, only normal pain from the operation." He signed her release form that day, and Sara and her baby went home.

On October 7, Josef called Dr. Jamal's office. "My wife is having severe stomach and abdominal pain. She needs to see you."

The doctor responded, "I'm sorry there are no appointments available. I can't see her today or tomorrow, but I can schedule her for an appointment on the tenth of October."

Since this was Sara's first baby, she didn't know if this pain was abnormal and the medical staff made her feel that it was a normal c-section pain so she shouldn't go to the emergency room.

The next day, Josef tried to phone Sara from his office but no one answered. Next, he called my husband because Bandar's office was closer to their home and pled, "Please go to my house as quickly as possible and check on Sara. She is not answering the phone."

When my husband arrived at Sara's house, he continuously rang the bell but no one answered. He heard the baby crying. Bandar broke the window and he jumped inside the house. When he ran to Sara's room, he found her unconscious and not breathing. He called 911 asking for help. When the emergency ambulance staff arrived, they told Bandar, "Sorry, Sara died over an hour ago."

Fifteen minutes later Josef arrived and saw Sara in the ambulance. With tears in his eyes, he asked his brother, "What is wrong with Sara?"

"I'm sorry. Sara is dead."

Josef learned the cause of death two weeks later, but he was shocked when he read the autopsy report. The report stated, "The surgeon, Dr. Jamal, who delivered the baby negligently left a medical tool inside the mother after he cut the umbilical cord. This failure caused blood intoxication, and a blood clot led to the death of the patient."

When Josef questioned hospital employees, he learned that Dr. Jamal was not a member of the hospital's medical staff, but he had a connection as his wife was the hospital's dentist. Josef also ascertained that the doctor was not authorized to perform any medical procedures in Saudi Arabia because he held a visitor visa. After more investigations, Josef found out that his wife's death was not Dr. Jamal's first negligence case. He had actually caused a number of severe problems and was ordered not to perform any medical work in any hospital in Saudi Arabia.

When Josef learned about Dr. Jamal, he started to look for a lawyer to sue the hospital. Josef didn't want any money, but he wanted the doctor and the hospital's manager to be punished for killing his wife.

The hospital director, Dr. Tariq, testified that he knew that doctors should not practice at the hospital without employment contracts. He emphasized that Dr. Jamal was qualified professionally to do various operations. He thought that no one should be held accountable for any possible negligence or malpractice.

Dr. Tariq added, "There are thousands of physicians working in hospitals in Saudi Arabia without a license or proper documents. But since the demand for medical staff is high in the obstetrics department, there are no proper procedures to make sure that everything is run correctly." He continued, "Dr. Jamal has been working for Albayan Hospital for over a year. He delivered over 120 babies. He only killed one person which is not a big problem. So what if Dr. Jamal doesn't have any contract with this hospital or any other hospital? There are many doctors who have their license and a contract, and they make similar errors. These mistakes happen everywhere. Why are you making this such a big deal?"

After nearly three months of hearings, deliberations, proceedings and investigation, the Ministry of Health concluded that the hospital was negligent. The case was further studied to determine the hospital's punishment. The Ministry of Health's committee submitted its findings and recommendations which called for closing that hospital's operating room and fining the doctor and the hospital one million Riyals. Finally, their report ordered that Dr. Jamal be deported and prohibited from returning to Saudi Arabia.

I wish I could tell the Dr. Jamal and Dr. Tariq one last thing, "The life of my closest friend is a very big deal." ✧

Faten Hamam is from Jeddah, Saudi Arabia. She graduated from King Abdullaziz University with a major in accounting. Currently, she lives in Miami with her husband and is earning her Master's degree in Health Service Administration at Barry University.

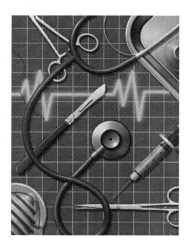

No Es Gran Problema

By Faten Hamam
Traducido por Frank Menendez y Francisco Menendez

Era 08 de octubre de 2008, yo había entrado a mi oficina en Jeddah, Arabia Saudita, cuando mi teléfono celular empezó a sonar sin detenerse. Pensé si debía responder a aquella llamada o no. En eso, mi amigo entró a la oficina con una mirada de preocupación en su rostro y me dijo: "Es su marido, Bandar, y dice que es urgente ".

Cogí el auricular y escuché la voz de mi marido. En su tono de voz me percaté de que algo terrible había pasado. Con voz temblorosa, me susurró, "Sara murió."

Mi corazón dio un vuelco. Con aquella noticia empezaba una pesadilla de la que no podía despertar. Me quedé sin habla por largo rato. Mis palabras definitivamente se negaban a salir de mi boca. Por último, mi marido me dijo: "Estaré en casa dentro de poco."

Al colgar el teléfono, traté de mantener la calma. Estaba en shock. No podía creer que Sara hubiera muerto. Éramos como hermanas y, de hecho, ella era mi cuñada. Sara fue quien me presentó a mi marido. Ambas habíamos asistido juntas a la universidad.

Aquella tragedia acababa de traumatizar tanto a mi marido como a mí.

Sara murió por complicaciones tras el parto. Su bebé nunca conocería a su madre por causa de un error médico.

La tragedia de Sara comenzó el 2 de octubre a las 2:15 am, cuando ella despertó experimentado algo extraño y que nunca antes había sentido. En aquella ocasión, Sara despertó a su esposo, Josef, y le hizo saber que ella temía de que algo andara mal con su embarazo. Este era el primer bebé de Sara, y ambos se sentían muy felices y emocionados de poder ser padres. Cuando él llamó al servicio de emergencias, explicó: "Mi esposa está embarazada con ocho meses y está sintiendo los dolores del parto. Por favor, venga tan rápido como puedan!" La ambulancia llegó a los quince minutos y un paramédico comprobó que Sara iba a tener un bebé. La llevaron al hospital más cercano. Mi marido le aconsejó a Josef que llamara a la madre de Sara para que también fuera al hospital.

Una enfermera vino a las 3.00 am y llevó a Sara a la sala de partos para prepararla, mientras que Josef seguía en la recepción del hospital llenando los papeles. El resto de la familia llegó un poco después. Josef se apresuró a entrar en la sala de parto para estar al lado de su esposa. Un par de horas más tarde, Josef regresó a la sala de espera donde estabamos todos nosotros y nos informó: "Acabo de hablar con el doctor Jamal y él cree que Sara no está dilatando lo suficiente, así es que el considera que Sara necesita una cesárea".

A las 8:00 AM, Josef volvió de nuevo a la sala de espera y exclamó: "Sara dio a luz a una niña muy hermosa. Ya la operación ha terminado pero Sara sigue inconsciente. "

A las 10:30 AM, Sara y su hija ya estaban en su habitación cuando Sara finalmente se despertó rodeada de familiares y amigos: en eso, todos empezaron a felicitarla. "Su nombre es Sereen", dijo Sara. La madre de Sara empezó a darle algunos consejos sobre cómo criar a su bebé y lo que debía y no debía hacer.

El 6 de octubre, el Dr. Jamal visitó a Sara. Ella, quejándose, le dijo: "Doctor, todavía tengo un dolor muy fuerte".

El médico le respondió: "No es nada grave, sólo el dolor normal de la operación." Y con la misma, el doctor Jamal firmó el alta médica y a los dos los mandó a casa.

El 7 de octubre, Josef llamó a la consulta del Dr. Jamal: "Doctor, Sara mi esposa está teniendo problemas en el estómago y también tiene dolor abdominal. Ella necesita que usted la vea."

El médico le respondió: "Lo siento, no hay citas disponibles. No puedo verla ni hoy ni mañana, pero sí le puedo hacerle una cita para el diez de Octubre ".

Ya que este era el primer bebé de Sara, ella no entendía nada sobre aquella clase de dolores y malestares, por otra parte, el personal médico la había hecho creer que todos aquellos malestares eran normales y fruto de la cesárea, y que por lo tanto, Sara no debía preocuparse y tampoco ir a la sala de emergencias.

Al día siguiente, cuando Josef había intentado hablar por teléfono con Sara pero sin conseguirlo, él decidió llamar a nuestra oficina. Ya que nuestra oficina estaba más cerca de la casa de Sara, Josef llamó a mi marido y le suplicó: "Por favor, vayan a mi casa lo más rápido posible porque algo tiene que estar pasando con Sara, ella no responde el teléfono. "

Cuando mi marido llegó a casa de Sara, tocó continuamente el timbre pero nadie respondía. Cuando Bandar oyó el llanto del bebé, no esperó más para romper la ventana y enseguida salto dentro de la casa. Al llegar a la habitación de Sara, la encontró inconsciente y le pareció que ella no respiraba. Bandar llamó al servicio de emergencias para pedir ayuda. Cuando el personal de la ambulancia se presentó, le afirmaron a Bandar: "Sí, ella murió ya hace más de una hora."

Quince minutos más tarde, Josef llegó y vio a Sara en la ambulancia. Con lágrimas en los ojos, le preguntó a su hermano, "¿Qué ha pasado?"

"Lo siento. Sara ha muerto."

Dos semanas más tarde, Josef, aún sin entender la causa de aquella muerte, se sorprendió al leer el informe de la autopsia. El informe declaraba: "El cirujano, el doctor Jamal, quien atendió el parto, después de cortar el condón umbilical, en un acto de suma negligencia, dejó un instrumento médico dentro del cuerpo de la paciente. Este grave error provocó una intoxicación masiva en la sangre y provocó un cuágulo que causó una muerte inmediata."

Cuando Josef habló con los empleados del hospital, se enteró de que el doctor Jamal no era miembro del personal médico del hospital, si acaso, el doctor Jamal, ya que su esposa era dentista de aquel hospital, tenía alguna que otra conexión allí. Josef también pudo comprobar que el susudicho doctor Jamal no estaba autorizado para llevar a cabo ciertos procedimientos médicos en Arabia Saudita, debido a que él estaba en aquel país con una visa de visitante. Después de hacer más investigaciones, Josef descubrió que la muerte de su esposa no había sido la primera negligencia de aquel supuesto doctor, sino que él había causado más llantos y angustias con sus prácticas, y por lo cual, ya se le habían puesto varias restriciones a su labor en Arabia Saudita.

Cuando Josef supo todas aquellas duras y tristes verdades sobre el Dr. Jamal, comenzó a buscar a un abogado para demandar al hospital. Josef no quería dinero, sino que quería que aquel individuo y el director del hospital fueran castigados por haber matado a su buena esposa Sara.

El director del hospital, el doctor Tariq, cuando le tocó testificar, dijo que, a pesar de que él sabía que los médicos ejercían en su hospital sin contrato de trabajo, hizo hincapié en que el doctor Jamal había sido calificado profesionalmente para hacer diversas operaciones, y alegó que nadie debía ser considerado responsable de cualquier posible negligencia o mala práctica que hubiera ocurrido en su hospital.

El doctor Tariq añadió: "Hay miles de médicos que trabajan en los hospitales en Arabia Saudita sin licencia o documentos adecuados. Pero ya que la demanda de personal médico es elevada, sobretodo en el departamento de obstetricia, no existen procedimientos adecuados para asegurarse de que todo se ejecute correctamente. " Y continuó: "El doctor Jamal ha estado trabajando para Albayan hospital durante más de un año. Asistió el parto de más de 120 bebés, y que haya matado a alguna persona, eso no es un gran problema. Si el doctor Jamal no tiene contrato con el hospital o con cualquier otro hospital, eso no es un gran problema. Hay muchos médicos que tienen su licencia y un contrato, y también cometen errores similares. Estos errores ocurren en todos lados, ¿por qué tienen qué ser tan importantes en este hospital? "

Después de casi tres meses de audiencias, de deliberaciones y de seguir procedimientos e investigaciones, el Ministerio de Salud

había llegado a la conclusión de que el hospital había actuado neg-
ligentemente. El caso fue estudiado a fondo para determinar qué
castigo imponerle al hospital. Un comité del Ministerio de Salud presentó sus conclusiones y recomendaciones y en las que se pedía el
cierre de los quirófanos del hospital, además de que exigía multar
a algunos médicos y al propio hospital por un millón de riales. Por
último, en aquel informe se ordenó que el doctor Jamal fuera de-
portado y de que se le prohibiera regresar a Arabia Saudita.

Al final, me hubiera gustado decirle al doctor Jamal y al doctor
Tariq una última cosa: "Que la vida de mi mejor amigo tiene un
valor muy grande." ☀

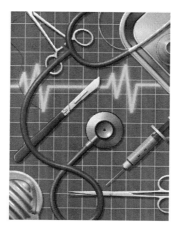

Se pa yon gwo zafè

Se Faten Hamam ki ekri istwa sa a
Translation: Roland Pierre

Se te 8 oktòb, 2008, mwen te nan biwo mwen nan Jeddah peyi Saudi Arabia lè ke mwen tande telefòn mwen ap sonnen san rete. Mwen mande zanmi mwen pou reponn telefòn la. Zanmi mwen a antre nan biwo a ak figi li ki te montre ke li te gen yon bagay ki te ap trakase li. Li di, "Se mari ou, Bandar. Li di se yon ijans."

Mwen pran telefòn la epi mwen tande vwa mari mwen. Sou son vwa li mwen konnen ke te gen yon bagay grav ki te ap pase. Nan yon vwa ki te ap tranble li di mwen tou ba, "Sara mouri Jodi a."

Se te tankou kè mwen te tonbe atè. Se te yon move rèv kote ke mwen te vle reveye. Mwen pa te ka pale. Okenn mote refize sòt nan bouch mwen. Alafen mwen sèlman di, "Map vinn lakay la touswit."

Lè ke mwen te ap fèmen telefòn la mwen te eseye rete kalm. Mwen te fè sezisman. Mwen pa te vle kwè ke Sara te mouri. Nou te tankou de sè, men anverite Sara pa te sè mwen li se te bèl sè mwen. Se li menm ki te fè mwen rankontre ak mari mwen. Nou te ale nan inivèsite ansanb. Lanmò sa se te yon trajedi ki te boulvèse mari mwen ak mwen menm anpil.

Sara te mouri paske li te fè pwoblèm apre ke li te finn akouche pitit li a. Ti pitit li a pap janm konnen manman li paske gen yon doktè ki te fè yon erè sou manman li.

Trajedi Sara a te kòmanse jou ki te 2 Oktòb a dezè kenz di maten lè ke li te leve epi ke li te santi yon bagay dwòl ke li pa te janm santi avan. Sara te leve mari li ki rele Joseph epi li di li kijan ke li te santi kò li. Tou le de te gen laperèz paske yo te kwè ke te gen yon bagy mal ki te ap pase ak ti bebe nan vant li a. Se te premye fwa ke Sara te ansent epi li menm ak mari li te tèlman kontan paske yo te ap pral vini paran yon ti moun.Joseph rele 911 epi li eksplike yo «Madanm mwen ansent 8 mwa epi li genyen anpil doulè. Tanpri vini pi vit ke nou kapab!"

Apre kenz minit, yon anbilans te rive epi paramredik yo te di, "Sara pral akouche ti bebe a. Nou ap mennen li nan lopital ki pi pre nou a." Josef te rele manman Sara, paran pa li yo epi mari pa mwen pou di yo pou tout moun rankontre nan lopital la.

Vè twazè, yon enfimyè vini epi li pouse charyot Sara te sou li a al nan sal akouchman pou yo te prepare li pandan ke Joseph te ap ranpli papye nan biwo pou anrejistre moun nan. Nou te ap rive lopital yon ti moman apre. Joseph te kouri al nan sal akouchman a pou li te avèk madanm li. Kèk è de tan apre joseph antre nan sal pou moun tann la epi li di nou «Mwen fèk pale ak Doktè Jamal ki deside ke travay akouchman Sara pa te ap mache vit ase, se pousa ke li te bezwen fè yon akouchman sezaryèn"

A 8 è dimaten, Joseph soti epi li di ak kè kontan «Sara fèk fè yon bèl pitit fi. Je li poko klè apre operasyon a."

Vè 10:30 di maten Sara ak pitit la te nan chanb lopital la lè sa anfen je li te klè epi tout moun te ap fè li konpliman. «Non li se Sereen" Sara te di avèk anpil lakontantman. Manman Sara te kòmanse ap ba li konsèy sou ki jan pou li leve timoun nan epi ap di li tout sa ke li dwe fè ak sa ke li pa dwe fè.

Le 6 Oktòb, Doktè Jamal te pase pou li tcheke Sara. Li te ap plenyen ba li «Mwen genyen doulè ki fò anpil"

Doktè a te reponn li «Se pa anyen serye, se doulè nòmal moun genyen lè yo fè operasyon" Li siyen papye lopital pou ke Sara kab ale lakay li epi jou sa aSara ale lakay li ak ti bebe a.

Le 7 Oktòb, Joseph rele klinik doktè Jamal la li di «Madanm mwen genyen gwo doulè nan vant li ak anba tivant li. Li bezwen wè ak ou"

Doktè a reponn li «Mwen regrèt pa gen randevou ki disponib. Mwen pa kab wè li jodi a oswa demen men mwen kab fè yon randevou pou le dis Oktòb."

Kòm se te premye pitit Sara, li pa te konnen si doulè a pa te nòmal epi moun ki te ap swanye li yo te fè li konprann ke se te doulè nòmal lè moun fè sezaryèn epi kidonk ke li pa te bezwen ale nan sal ijans.

Jou anapre a, pandan ke Joseph te nan biwo li li eseye rele madanm li, men li pa te reponn telefòn la. Apre sa a li rele biwo Bandar la paske li te pi pre lakay li a lè sa a li te lapryè li «Tanpri ale lakay la pi vit ke ou kapab epi tcheke Sara. Li pa reponn telefòn la."

Lè ke mari mwen te rive kay Sara a eke li te ap peze sonèt nan pòt la san rete san ke pèsonn pa te reponn.Li tande tibebe a ap krye. Lè sa a, Bandar te kraze yon fenèt epi li te vole antre nan kay la. Lè ke li te kouri ale nan chanb Sara a, li te jwenn li san konesans epi li pate ap respire. Li te rele 911 pou mande yo sekou. Lè ekip moun ki travay nan anbilans la te rive yo te di Bandar «Nou regrèt, Sara te mouri te gen yon è detan."

Kenz minit apre joseph rive epi li wè Sara nan anbilans la . Ak dlo nan je li li mande frè Sara a «Sa Sara genyen?"

«Mwen regrèt Sara mouri"

Se te de semèn apre ke joseph te vinn konnen sa ki te tiye Sara men li te fè sezisman lè ke li te li rapò otopsi a. Rapò a te di «Doktè chirijyen ki te fè operasyon akouchman a te fè neglijans li te kite yon zouti andedan fanm ke li te akouche a lè ke li te koupe kòd lonbrit ti moun nan. Zouti sa a ke yo pa te retire a te lakòz ke san li te anpwazonnen, epi boul san kaye te lakòz ke patyan a te mouri."

Lè ke Joseph te ap mande anplwaye lopital yo keksyon li te vinn konnen ke Doktè Jamal pat fè pati nan doktè ki travay nan lopital la, men ke li te fè akouchman la paske li te rsevwa favè akòz madanm li se te dantist nan lopital la. Joseph vinn konnen trè byen ke doktè a pa te gen dwa travay sou malad nan peyi Saudi Arabia paske se sèlman yon viza pou moun ki ap vizite peyi a ke li te genyen. Apre ke li fè lòt envestigasyon, joseph vinn konnnen ke lanmò madanm li a se pa te premye ka moun ki te mouri akòz neglijans doktè sa a. Li vinn konnen ke doktè a te lakòz anpil pwoblèm grav epi ke akòz tout move zak sa yo yo te ba li lòd pou li pa travay kom doktè nan okenn lopital nan Saudi Arabia.

Lè ke Joseph vinn konnen tout zak doktè Jamal, li komanse chèche yon avoka pou li rele lopital la lajistis sa yo rele su moun nan. Joseph pa te ap chèche jwen lajan men li te vle pini doktè a ak administratè lopital la pou madanm li yo te tiye a.

Doktè Tariq ki te direktè lopital la te temwanye ke li te konnen ke yon doktè ki pa te gen kontra pou li te travay nan lopital la pa te dwe ap travay epi swanye malad. Li fè remake ke doktè Jamal se te yon pwofesyonèl ki te byen prepare pou li fè anpil kalite operasyon. Li di ke okenn moun pa te dwe jwen kondanasyon paske te gen yon neglijans medikal ki ta sipoze te fèt.

Doktè Tariq te di «Gen plis ke mil doktè ki ap travay nan Saudi Arabia san ke yo pa gen lisans pou travay kòm doktè oswa gen papye yo ki annòd. Men kòm yo bezwen doktè anpil nan branch ki fè akouchman yo rele obstetrik pa gen mwayen pou yo asire yo ke tout bagay ap mache kòm sa dwatèt. Li kontinye «Doktè Jamal gen ennan ke li ap travay ak lopital Albayan. Li akouche plis ke 120 tibebe. Li tiye yon sèl moun se pa yon gwo zafè. Ki pwoblèm si doktè Jamal pa gen kontra ak lopital mwen a oswa lòt lopital? Gen plizyè doktè ki gen lisans yo epi ki gen kontra epi ki fè menm erè sa yo. Erè sa yo rive nenpòt ki kote. Pou kisa nou vle fè ka sa a yon gwo zafè?"

Apre prèske twa mwa ap tande temwen, ap delibere, ap fè prosè a, ap fè envestigasyon, Ministè Lasante a te jwen ke lopital la te fè neglijans. Yo te etidye ka Sara a pi plis pou yo te konnen ki kalite pinisyon pou yo te bay lopital la. Komite Ministè Lasante te bay sa ke li te jwen apre yo etidye ka a epi li te bay sa ke li te rekòmande ki se te pou fèmen sal operasyon lopital la epi fè doktè ak lopital la peye yon milyon Riyals. Alafen nan rapò yo, yo te rekòmande pou ke yo depòte doktè Jamal epi bay lòd pou li pa janmen tounen nan peyi Saudi Arabia.

Mwen swete mwen te kab di doktè Jamal ak doktè Tariq yon dènye bagay; "Lavi pi bon zanmi mwen se yon gwo zafè." ※

Faten Hamam se yon moun ki soti nan Jeddah, nan peyi Saudi Arabia. Li diplome nan inivèsite King Abdullaziz University la li te espesyalize li nan kontabilite. Kounyea li ap viv nan Miami ak mari li epi li ap etidye pou li gen mastè li nan Sèvis Administrasyon Lasante nan inivèsite Barry University.

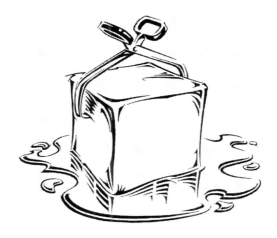

Keeping it on Ice

By Carolyn Tejirian

My pediatric rotation started with some of the sickest children I had ever encountered. During my first two weeks on the wards, I was assigned to hematology/oncology. Although I had several patients who were infants and toddlers - a joy for a medical student to play with - my most memorable patient was a seventeen year-old on the brink of his manhood. In fact, he was a large teenager. He played linebacker on his high school football team. Despite his physical appearance, he was very much a teenager. He answered the most open-ended of questions with either a shrug or a monosyllabic word, and his hobbies included all things football and video games (ideally, video games about football).

One day, while living in his small town, he started getting headaches. These headaches started each morning as a dull pain, and over the course of the day became unbearable. Soon he developed double vision, and subsequently was diagnosed with a brain tumor.

His family lived in a small rural town several hundred miles away from the hospital. His father worked at home while his mother stayed with her sick son in the hospital.

I met him following his first operation to remove as much of the tumor as possible. We were about to start his chemo therapy and radiation treatment. On my first day with this patient the oncologist I was working under brought up a topic I never thought I would encounter in pediatrics. Addressing both our young patient and his mother, she said, "We are about to start an aggressive treatment plan, which in addition to battling the cancer, may have lasting effects. As we discussed last time, the treatment may affect your ability to have children in the future. Have you given any thought to banking your sperm?"

Our young patient was very quiet, his mother answered, "Yes, we discussed it. Even though our insurance does not cover it, we're willing to pay the two hundred and fifty dollars a year to keep his sperm on ice."

As the details of sperm banking were discussed: when, where and how a deposit would be made, my poor patient kept quietly staring down at his lap, clearly wishing the earth would open up and swallow him whole. To make matters worse, everyone responsible for the care of our patient was female: the oncologist, the pediatric resident, the nurse, the social worker, his mother, and me – all female.

Medical students do not make the final decision about the treatment plan for our patients. We can recommend what we think is the best course of action and discuss it with residents and attending physicians, which is how we learn. We are however, involved in all aspects of our patient's care. This is how I ended up on the phone with the sperm bank and the social worker trying to make an appointment for our patient. The plan was to discharge the patient, give him and his mother a cab voucher to take them to the sperm bank; he would make the deposit, then take a cab back, and be readmitted into the hospital.

"We really can't accept him here," explained the sperm bank lady. "We don't want the legal responsibility for someone who should still be in the hospital. We can give you a sample cup. As soon as you have the sample, it is good for two hours before we have to freeze it. Just bring it to our clinic."

The social worker agreed. "Legally the hospital could be in trouble if anything were to happen to our patient" she clarified. Our patient, by this point, was wheelchair bound because the double vision made walking too difficult.

"Well, that saves us the hassle of getting to the sperm bank," I said. "Can't we just get him to make the deposit in his room, and then have his mother carry it to the bank?"

"Nope," the social worker shook her head. "We don't do anything that might sound painful in the patient's room on the pediatric floor, and this would count as painfully awkward." I nodded in agreement.

A good social worker suggested that I call the urology department. They didn't do sperm banking but they might have the facilities to make the deposit. I immediately called down to their clinic, and they agreed. Later that afternoon, I placed my patient in a wheelchair, and took him to the urology clinic. In the elevator, I felt awkward. I couldn't imagine what my patient was feeling. "Are you clear with the plan and what you're about to do?" I asked. He nodded. That is all we said to each other. In hind sight, I should have said more.

I handed off his wheelchair to the nurse in urology and took a seat in the waiting room. An hour later the nurse came back shacking sadly. "He wasn't successful, and we need the room for another patient." So I wheeled my patient back to his room.

Later that afternoon, the oncologist went to visit him. She leaned in closely and with a conspiratorial whisper asked, "So, did they give you any good girly magazines?"

While staring intently at his feet, he answered in a whisper, "No."

When we left his room, the cancer doctor turned to me, "Carolyn, go back to urology and find out what happened. Also call the sperm bank again. If I have to drive him there myself, I will. We are running out of time. We start his therapy tomorrow."

Back in urology I asked the nurse about any aids that were provided. "No, we didn't give him anything," she explained. "When we handed him the consent form to sign he really didn't seem to understand it, so we didn't think a magazine would help."

"He has terrible double vision," I exclaimed. "He is not really fond of his eye patch. Although he can't read, I'm sure he can look at pictures of big breasts." I was done being awkward. "If we bring him back tomorrow, what can you offer?" She pointed to two, tattered, twenty-year old copies of Playboy. I grabbed some latex gloves and flipped through them. The magazines were older than my patient, and featured big-haired, women wearing lingerie that was no longer in style. Sure, a naked woman is a naked woman, but we only had one more chance at this.

Next, I called the sperm bank back. "We just don't have the facilities here for our patient to make the deposit," I explained. "All we can do is put him in a sterile exam room in the urology clinic. We don't have any magazines or DVDs. We start treatment tomorrow, and this will affect the rest of his life." The woman at the bank was not sympathetic. "We don't have a room either. We have a closet with a plastic chair and sink."

"Really?" I asked. "I always imagined it the way it's portrayed on TV, with a man being handed a stack of magazines and videos."

"Not even close," she retorted. "Most of our clients take a sterile cup home and bring it back."

I hung up thinking, you learn something new everyday. Today I was learning plenty.

I returned to the attending oncologist and told her the situation.

"Alright, a new game plan is needed," she stated with resolve. "We need to put together a pediatric department sperm donation kit. Who wants to do it?"

"This is my patient," I stated. "I'll do it."

That night, I left the hospital with a mission. I had never purchased explicitly sexual materials before, so I wasn't really sure where to buy it. As far and I was concerned, this stuff came from the internet. I headed to the part of town with all the strip clubs and the Hustler store. I bee-lined for the magazine section. Given the urology department's track record, I was not sure they owned a DVD player.

The next day, I showed up at the hospital with my sperm donation kit. It included three magazines and two DVDs all concealed in a large, unmarked manila envelope. My attending resident told me the patient was already down in urology. "Doc, here is the kit." We thought the patient would be more comfortable if a male handed him this material.

He couldn't stop smiling. "I can't believe you did this," he said I handed him the kit. "It is the ultimate scut work. You didn't have to do it." Scut work is medical jargon for the multitude of busy work that is done in a hospital. As a general rule, this is minimized for medical students whose primary objective is to learn medicine. "I even called some of my buddies from med school in New York and told them what you were doing."

"Someone had to do it," I responded grinning. "I feel so bad for him. This is so amazingly awkward." I admit that I was glad to be handing off this responsibility, temporarily, to someone else. We knew that it had to get done this morning because therapy was scheduled to start in the afternoon.

Later, the hematology/oncology team was meeting in the small conference room where we were discussing all of our patients when a nurse poked her head in and declared, "Success! He did it!" The reaction in the room was a mix between cheering and sighs of relief. The nurse, smiling, added "the urology department wanted to know if they could keep the kit."

"Hell no," came the immediate response from my attending. "Did you grab it back? We are going to use this for future pediatric patients who need to bank their sperm."

"Of course," stated the nurse with confidence. "They can make their own kit."

The motivating factor for many who go into medicine, not just physicians but any aspect of medicine is the chance to make a lasting and positive contribution to someone's life, whether it is to treat an illness or just make life a little easier. I'd like to think that my team (the physicians, the nurses, the social worker, and me, the student) went beyond the disease and treated the person. Although I am sure that our seventeen-year old patient still wishes that the earth had swallowed him whole, someday, when he has beat his cancer and is an adult, he will be able to put our efforts to good use and start a family. ⚕

Carolyn Tejirian is a first-year resident in Family Medicine at the University of New Mexico in Albuquerque, New Mexico. She is a graduate of Tulane University Medical School.

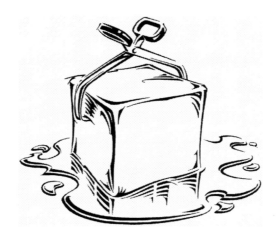

Manténiendolo
en Hielo

By Carolyn Tejirian
Traducido por Frank Menendez y Francisco Menendez

Mi turno de pediatría se inició con algunos de los niños más enfermos que yo había tratado en toda mi vida. Durante mis primeras dos semanas en las sala, me asignaron a hematología-oncología. A pesar de que tenía varios pacientes que eran bebés y niños pequeños, —algo alegre para un estudiante de medicina ya que podría jugar con ellos— mi paciente más memorable fue un joven de diecisiete años de edad, ya al borde de la adultez. De hecho, él era un adolescente de gran estatura física. Él había jugado como defensa de su equipo de fútbol de la escuela. Pero a pesar de su fuerte apariencia física, era un adolescente. Él respondía a las más difíciles de las preguntas con un encogimiento de hombros o un monosílabo; sus pasatiempos estaban relacionados con el fútbol, hasta los videojuegos.

Un día, mientras vivía en su pequeño pueblo, él empezó a tener dolores de cabeza. Estos dolores que sentía cada mañana comenzaron siendo un dolor mínimo, y durante el día se hacían insoportables. Bastante pronto, comenzó a ver doble; y posteriormente se le diagnosticó un tumor cerebral.

Su familia vivía en un pequeño pueblo rural a varios cientos de kilómetros de distancia del hospital. Su padre trabajaba en la casa mientras que la madre se quedaba con el hijo enfermo en el hospital.

Lo conocí después de la primera operación que trato de extirparle el tumor: estábamos a punto de comenzar el tratamiento de quimioterapia y radioterapia. En mi primer día con este paciente, la oncóloga, que trabajaba conmigo, inició un tema de conversación que nunca pensé encontrar en pediatría. Dirigiéndose tanto a nuestro paciente como a su madre, la oncóloga dijo: "Estamos a punto de comenzar un plan de tratamiento agresivo, que además de luchar contra el cáncer, puede tener efectos duraderos. Pero, tal y como hablamos la última vez, el tratamiento puede afectar su capacidad de tener hijos en el futuro. ¿Ha considerado la posibilidad de almacenar su esperma?"

Nuestro paciente joven se quedó callado, su madre respondió: "Sí, ya lo discutimos. A pesar de que nuestro seguro no lo cubre, estamos dispuestos a pagar los doscientos cincuenta dólares al año para mantener su esperma en el hielo."

Mientras los detalles de un banco de esperma se discutían: cuándo, dónde y cómo un depósito se podría hacer, mi pobre paciente se mantenía en silencio mirando hacia abajo, claramente deseando que la tierra se abriera y se lo tragara entero. Para empeorar las cosas, todos los responsables de su cuidado eran mujeres: la oncóloga, la residente de pediatría, la enfermera, la trabajadora social, su madre, y yo: todas éramos mujeres.

Los estudiantes de medicina no toman la decisión final sobre el plan de tratamiento de los pacientes. Podemos recomendar lo que pensamos es lo mejor y discutirlo con los residentes y los médicos, pues es la manera de aprender. Estamos, sin embargo, involucrados en todos los aspectos de la atención de nuestros pacientes. Por esa razón estaba en el teléfono con el banco de esperma y la trabajadora social, tratando de hacer una cita para nuestro paciente. Debíamos darle un alta temporal, y pagarle el servicio de un taxi para que lo llevaran a un banco de esperma, y después que el paciente hiciera el depositó, regresaría al hospital en el mismo taxi.

"Realmente no podemos recibirlo aquí", explicó la señora del banco de esperma. "No queremos responsabilidad legal con alguien que todavía es su paciente en su hospital. Podemos darle una vasija y tan pronto como obtenga una muestra, que sirve por dos horas antes de congelarla, no las trae a nuestra clínica. "

La trabajadora social estaba de acuerdo. "Legalmente, el hospital podría estar en problemas si algo llegara a sucederle al paciente", aclaró. Nuestro paciente, ya en este momento, estaba en silla de ruedas debido a la dificultad de caminar ya que veía doble.

"Bien, eso nos ahorra la molestia del viaje al banco de esperma", le dije. "No podemos llevarlo a hacer el depósito en su habitación, y luego que su madre lo lleve al banco?"

"No", la trabajadora social sacudió la cabeza. "No haga nada en la habitación de pediatría, que pueda ser doloroso para él." Yo estaba de acuerdo en este aspecto.

La trabajadora social me sugirió que llamara al departamento de urología. Ellos no mantenían bancos de esperma, pero podrían tener las instalaciones para hacer el depósito. De inmediato llamé a la clínica, y ellos aceptaron. En la tarde, puse a mi paciente en una silla de ruedas, y lo llevé a la clínica. En el ascensor, me sentía incómoda. No me podía imaginar lo que mi paciente sentía. "¿Está usted claro con el plan y lo que va a hacer?", pregunté. Él asintió con la cabeza. Eso es todo lo que nos dijimos el uno al otro. En retrospectiva, yo debería haber dicho más.

Le pasé la silla de ruedas a la enfermera de urología y me senté en la sala de espera. Una hora más tarde la enfermera regresó triste. "Él no tuvo éxito, y necesitamos el espacio para otro paciente." Así que lleve mi paciente a su habitación.

Por la tarde, la oncóloga fue a visitarlo. Se acercó a él y con un susurro de conspiradora le preguntó: "¿no te dieron ninguna revista buena?"

Mientras miraba fijamente a sus pies, él contestó en un susurro: "No"

Cuando salimos de su habitación, el médico especialista en cáncer se volvió hacia mí "Carolyn, vuelve a urología y averigua lo que sucedió. También se debe consultar al banco de esperma de nuevo. Si tengo que conducirlo personalmente, lo haré. Queda poco tiempo. Mañana comenzamos el tratamiento".

De vuelta en urología le pregunté a la enfermera acerca de las ayudas que se le proporcionaron al paciente. "No, no les dimos nada", explicó. "Cuando le entregué el formulario de consentimiento para que lo firmara no parecía entenderlo, así que no creímos que una revista sería de ayuda."

"Él tiene visión doble", exclamé. "Él no está acostumbrado a tener un parche en el ojo. A pesar de que no puede leer, estoy segura de que puede ver fotos de pechos grandes." Yo empezaba a sentirme molesta ante tantas dificultades. "Si queremos traerlo de vuelta mañana, ¿qué le puedes ofrecer?" Ella señaló a dos viejas copias de Playboy. Cogí unos guantes de látex y pasé las páginas. Las revistas eran mas viejas que mi paciente, y mostraban mujeres con ropa interior que ya no estaba en estilo. Claro, una mujer desnuda es una mujer desnuda, pero sólo tenía una oportunidad más en esto.

A continuación, llamé al banco de esperma de vuelta. "Simplemente no contamos con las instalaciones aquí para que nuestro paciente hiciera el depósito," le expliqué. "Todo lo que podemos hacer es ponerlo en la consulta de urología. No tenemos ninguna revista o DVD. Debemos empezar el tratamiento mañana, pero antes debemos resolver lo de la esperma, si no lo conseguimos esto lo afectará el resto de su vida. "La mujer en el banco no era comprensiva. "Aquí tampoco tenemos una habitación. Tenemos un armario con una silla de plástico y un lavabo."

"¿En serio?", Pregunté. "Siempre me imaginé la forma en que todo esto aparece en la televisión, donde aparece un hombre al que se le daba una pila de revistas y videos."

"Ni siquiera cerca", replicó ella. "La mayoría de nuestros clientes se llevan a su hogar un recipiente estéril y los traen de vuelta."

Me quedé pensando, se aprende algo nuevo todos los días. Hoy estaba aprendiendo un montón.

Volví al oncóloga y le hable de la situación.

"Muy bien, necesitamos un plan nuevo", afirmó con decisión. "Tenemos nosotros mismos que resolver lo de la donación de espermatozoides. ¿Quién quiere participar?"

"Este es mi paciente", afirmé. "Yo lo haré."

Esa noche, salí del hospital con una misión. Yo nunca había comprado materiales explícitamente sexuales, así que no estaba muy segura de dónde comprarlos. Me dirigí a la parte de la ciudad donde están todos los clubes de striptease y la tienda Hustler. Dado el historial del Servicio de Urología, ni siquiera estaba segura si poseíamos un reproductor de DVD.

Al día siguiente, me presenté en el hospital con mi "kit de donación de esperma." Incluía tres revistas y dos DVD. Todo oculta en un sobre grande, sin marcas. El residente me dijo que el paciente estaba ya en urología. "Doctor, aquí está el material audiovisual." Pensábamos que el paciente estaría más cómodo si un hombre se lo entregaba.

No podía dejar de sonreír. "No puedo creer que hayas hecho esto", dijo. "Es el trabajo sucio. No tienes que hacerlo." Trabajo sucio es la jerga médica para la gran cantidad de trabajos ocupados que se lleva a cabo en un hospital. Como regla general, esto se reduce al mínimo para estudiantes de medicina, cuyo principal objetivo es aprender la medicina. "Incluso llamé a algunos de mis compañeros de la escuela de medicina en Nueva York y les dije lo que estaba haciendo."

"Alguien tenía que hacerlo", le respondí con una sonrisa. "Me siento muy mal por él. Esto es tan increíblemente torpe. "Tengo que reconocer que me alegré dándole esta responsabilidad, aunque sea temporal, a otra persona. Sabíamos que teníamos que conseguirlo antes del próximo día porque el tratamiento iba a comenzar en la tarde.

Esa tarde, el equipo de hematología-oncología se reunió en la pequeña sala de conferencias cuando una enfermera asomó la cabeza y declaró: "!Éxito! ¡Él lo hizo! "La reacción en la sala fue de una mezcla de aplausos y suspiros de alivio. La enfermera, sonriendo, añadió: "el servicio de urología quería saber si podía quedarse con el kit."

"Por supuesto que no", fue la respuesta inmediata de mi asistente. "¿Lo agarrastes de nuevo? Vamos a usar esto para futuros pacientes pediátricos que necesiten depositar su esperma. "

"Por supuesto", dijo la enfermera con confianza. "Ellos pueden hacer su propio equipo."

El factor de motivación para muchos de los que van a la medicina, no sólo médicos, sino a cualquier campo de la medicina, es la oportunidad de hacer una contribución duradera y positiva a la vida de alguien, ya sea para tratar una enfermedad o simplemente hacer la vida un poco más fácil. Me gustaría pensar que mi equipo (los médicos, las enfermeras, la trabajador social, y para mí, la estudiante) aquello fue más allá de la enfermedad, y pudieron tratar a la persona. Aunque estoy segura de que nuestro paciente de diecisiete años de edad todavía desea que la tierra se lo trague. Pero, algún día, cuando haya ganado la batalla contra el cáncer y sea un adulto, será capaz de aprovechar nuestros esfuerzos para formar una familia. ☼

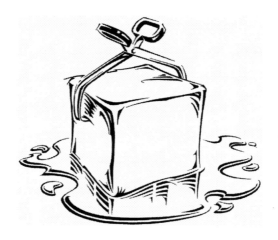

Pou kenbe li nan glas

Se Carolyn Tejirian ki ekri istwa sa a
Translation Roland Pierre

Rotasyon mwen nan sèvis pedyatri lopital la te kòmanse ak timoun ki pi malad ke mwen te janm rankontre nan lavi mwen. Pandan de premye semenn ke mwen te nan sal, la yo te mete mwen travay nan ematoloji onkoloji sèvis ki okipe maladi nan san ak kansè.

Menm ke mwen te genyen plizyè patyan ki te ti moun piti, sa ki pote kè kontan pou ton moun ki ap etidye doktè lè ke li kapab jwe ak yo. Men malad ke mwen pi sonje se yon jenn gason ki te gen disètan e ki te preske gran moun. An verite se te yon jenn gason ki, te byen grandi. Li te jwe foutbòl ameriken nan lekòl segondè kote li te ale a epi se li ki te linebacker sa vle di aryè nan ekip la. Malgre jan ke li te byen grandi a li se te vreman tankou yon jenn gason ki poko granmoun sa yo rele adolesan yo, tout keksyon yo te mande li ki te merite pou li bay yon repons ak eksplikasyon li te konn reponn ak zepòl li ke li te monte oswa ak yon sèl mo. Sa li te renmen fè pou lwazi li se te jwe foutbòl ameriken epi jwe jwèt video ki te sou zafè foutbòl.

Yon jou pandan ke li te ap viv nan ti vil li a li te kòmanse gen maltèt. Maltèt sa yo te komanse chak maten ak yon doulè ki te tou piti ki te li te vinn paka sipote lè ke jounen tap fini. Apre ke yon ti tan te finn pase, li te vinn wè doub epi apre yo te vinn fè dyagnostik ke li te gen yon timè nan tèt li.

Fanmi jenn gason sa a te ap viv nan yon ti vil nan zòn riral ki te tabli plizyè mil distans ak lopital la. Papa li te ap travay lakay li pandan ke manman li te rete ak pitit gason li a ki te malad nan lopital la.

Mwen te kontre ak jenn gason malad la apre premye operasyon yo te fè pou retire pi plis kantite timè yo te kapab nan sèvo li. Ekip doktè yo ta pral kòmanse bay jenn gason a tretman ak pwodyi chimik ak reyon pou tiye selil ki te gen kansè yo.

Nan premye jou ak patyan a onkolojist la kidonk doktè ki trete maladi kansè a te vinn ak yon koze ke mwen pa te janm kè ke mwen ta tande nan sèvis pedyatri a. Lè ke li te ap pale ak jenn patyan ak manman li li te di "Nou pral fè yon trètman ki ap fò anpil kidonk yon tretman kraze zo ki anplis ke li ap konbat kansè a ap gen move konsekans ki ap dire pou tout tan sou lòt pati nan kò jenn gason a. Tankou nou te di ou dènye fwa a tretman kapab lakòz ke ou pa kapab fè pitit apre tretman a.Eske ou reflechi sou zafè pou ou mete jèm ou nan yon kote yo sere jèm gason yo rele labank?"

Jenn patyan a te rete san pale manman li te reponn, " wi nou te pale sou sa. Menm si asirans la pap peye labank la pou sere jèm jenn gason a nou dakò pou nou peye desan senkant dola pa an ke yo mande pou kenbe jèm li nan glas."

Kòm yo te ap diskite detay kijan sere jèm la nan labank la te ap fèt nou te pale sou ki kote, ki lè, epi kijan ke yo te ap ranmase jèm jenn gason a, pòv jenn gason te rete san pale ap gade jenou li, li te klè ke li te ap swete ke latè te louvri epi ke li te antre ladan li tout antye. Bagay yo te pi mal paske tout moun ki te reskonsab pou bay patyan a laswenyaj se te fi: doktè kansè a, doktè ki te rezidan nan pedyatri a, enfimyè a, travayè sosyal la, manman li epi mwen menm nou tout se te fanm.

Moun ki ap aprann doktè pa pran desizyon sou ki dènye plan ki pou fèt pou trete yon patyan. Nou menm etidyan doktè nou kalkile sa ki pi bon pou yon malad nou diskite li ak doktè rezidan a epi ak doktè ki reskonsab la epi se konsa ke nou aprann. Menm si nou pa fè desizyon sou tretman a nou la pou fè tout sa ke malad la bezwen lè ke yo ap trete li. Men sa ke yo te vle fè, yo te ap ba malad la pèmi-syon pou soti nan lopital la, bay manman li ak li yon papye ki te peye taxi pou yo epi voye yo nan labank ki kenbe jèm gason a; lè sa jenn gason a ta va bay jèm la nan labank la, lè li te fini bay jèm la li te ap pran yon lòt taxi pou li tounen lopital la, epi lopital la te ap fè li antre lopital kòm malad ankò.

"Nou pa kab aksepte li nan labank pou jèm la" te eksplike yon madam ki travay la.

"Nou pa kapab pran responsabilite pou yon moun ki dwe kouche lopital. Nou kapab ba ou yon bokal pou mete echantiyon jèm la. Menm moman ke ou gen echantiyon jèm la ou va pote li banou nan labank la pou nou jele li nan glas, echantiyon jèm la bon pandan dezè de tan apre ke moun nan mete li deyò annik pote li nan klinik la lè jenn gason a fini."

Travayè sosyal la te dakò "dapre lalwa lopital la te kapab nan pwoblèm si gen yon bagay ki rive patyan a." li ajoute. Lè sa a patyan a te ap deplase nan yon chèz woulant paske li te wè doub epi li te two difisil pou li mache.

Ebyen mwen di "sa ap epanye nou traka pou voye jenn gason a nan labank pou jèm la" "Eske nou pa kapab fè li bay jèm la nan chamb malad li a epi fè manman li pote echantiyon jèm la nan la-bank la" mwen te di.

Non travayè sosyal la di "Nou pa fè anyen ki parèt bay moun nan doulè nan chamb la lè moun nan nan sèvis pedyatri a, epi sa va parèt dwòl anpil" mwen sekwe tèt mwen pou mwen di ke mwen te dakò ak li.

Bon travayè sosyal la bay lide pou nou rele sèvis iroloji lopital la.Yo pa fè zafè mete jèm gason nan labank men yo te kapab gen kote pou moun nan mete echantiyon jèm la deyò. Menm moman a mwen rele klinik iroloji a epi yo te dakò. Vè pita nan apremidi, mwen mete patyan mwen a nan yon chèz woulant epi mwen mennen li nan klinik iroloji a. Nan asansè a mwen te santi ke mwen te dwòl. Mwen pa te kapab imajine ki sa ke patyan mwen a te santi "Eske ou kon-pran sa ke yo vle fè pou ou a, eske ou dakò ak sa ou pral fè a?" mwen te mande li. Li sekwe tèt li pou di mwen wi. Se sa sèlman ke yonn te di lòt. Lè ke mwen ap reflechi sou sa kounye a, mwen wè ke se pou mwen te di li plis ke sa a.

Mwen lonje chèz li a bay enfimyè nan sèvis iroloji a epi mwen chita sou yon chèz nan sal pou moun tann la. Yon è de tan apre enfimyè a tounen ak figi li byen chagren" Li pa reyisi bay echantiyon jèm la, epi nou bezwen chanb la pou yon lòt patyan" Kidonk mwen woule chèz la pou mwen mennen patyan a tounen nan chanb li.

Vè pita nan jou sa a, doktè ki trete kansè a te vini wè malad la.Li panche tou pre li epi nan yon ti vwa moun ki ap met tèt ansanb pou fè yon bagay li mande li " Alò yo te ba ou kèk bon ti revi dekòlte ki gen fi ladan yo?"

Pandan ke li te fè ekspre pou li fixe je li sou gade pye li li reponn tou ba, "Non"

Lè ke nou kite chanb malad la doktè kansè a vire gade mwen li di : " Carolyn,tounen ale nan iroloji epi cheche konnen sa ki te pase. Epi rele labank pou jèm gason a ankò.Si se pou mwen mete li nan oto pou mwen mennen li mwen menm mwen va fè sa.Nou pa gen anpil tan ki rete ankò.Nou ap komanse tretman a demen. "

Lè ke mwen retounen ale nan iroloji a mwen mande enfimyè a si yo te bay malad kèk bagay pou ede li mete jèm la deyò. Li esplike: "No nou pa te ba li anryen ditou.Lè ke nou te bali fòm pou li konsanti fè sa ke li te dwe fè a li te sanble ke li pa te twò konprann anyen, kidonk nou te kwè ke yon ti revi dekolte ak fi ladan li pa tap sèvi a anyen.

"Je li pa bon li wè doub " mwen eksplike enfimyè a .Li pa vreman renmen pansman ki sou je li a. Menm si li pa kab li mwen si ke li kapab gade foto fi ak gwo tete. Mwen te sispann jennen mwen di li "Si nou mennen li demen ki sa ke ou ap genyen pou ofri li?" Li lonje dwèt sou de vye kopi revi Playboy ki gen plis ke ventan e ki te finn dechèpiye. Mwen mete gan plastik nan men mwen epi mwen feyte revi yo. Revi yo te pi gran pase jenn gason a epi ladan yo se te fi ak gwo cheve ki te gen sou yo soutyen ak kilòt ki pat a la mòd ankò ki te genyen. Se vre ke yon fanm toutouni se yon fanm toutouni men kòm nou te rete sèlman yon chans pou sa mache mewen te dwe pou fè yon bagay.

Apre sa mwen rele labank pou jèm la ankò; "Nou pa gen bon kondisyon pou patyan a bay jèm la isit la nou gen yon chanb nan klinik iroloji a ki pa gen okenn dekorasyon ladan li nou pa gen revi dekolte oswa DVD. Nou ap kòmanse tretman a demen epi se yon bagay ki ap gen konsekans pou tout rès vi li." Fanm ki te ap travay nan labank jèm la pa te janti ditou li te reponn : "Nou pa gen chanb nonplis isit la. Nou gen yon klosèt, yon chèz an plastik, epi yon lavabo."

"Vreman" mwen te di li " Mwen te toujou konprann ke se menm jan yo montre sa nan television ke sa te ye ak yon pakèt revi dekolte epi video."

"Se pa sa ditou" li te reponn. "Laplipa klyan nou yo pran bokal pou mete echantiyon a epi yo pote li ale lakay yo epi lè ke yo fini yo pote li tounen ban nou."

Mwen fèmen telefòn la epi mwen te ap reflechi ke mwen aprann yon bagay chak jou. Jodi a mwen te ap aprann anpil.

Mwen tounen al jwen doktè ki okipe kansè e ki te reskonsab malad la epi mwen di li sa ki te ap pase a.

Li di ak konviksyon: " Se bon kounye a nou bezwen yon lòt plan. Nou bezwen mete sou pye yon twous zouti pou malad pedyatri by jèm yo. Ki moun ki vle okipe yo de sa."

"Se patyan mwen li ye mwen ap okipe mwen de sa" mwen reponn.

Jou swa sa a mwen kite lopital la ak yon misyon. Mwen pa te jan achte liv ak video dekolte avan sa mwen pa te konnen kote pou mwen te jwen yo pou mwen achte. Pou sa ki te konsène mwen kalite bagay sa yo se nan entènèt ke moun jwen yo. Mwen pran direksyon kote nan vil la ki te gen klèb kote moun ap dezabiye yo toutouni epi boutik ki vann bagay dekolte. Mwen pran wout pati ki vann revi yo. Pou jan ke depatman iroloji te pate gen anyen mwen pa te kwè ke yo te genyen yon aparèy pou jwe DVD.

Jou an apre a, mwen parèt nan lopital la ak twous zouti pou moun mete jèm li deyo. Li te gen ladan li twa revi dekolte ak de video tout sa byen kache nan yon gwo anvlòp jòn kip a te make anyen. Doktè rezidan a te di mwen ke patyan nou a te déjà desann nan iroloji. "Dòk men twous zouti a" Nou te kwè ke patyan a te ap pi alèz si se te yon gason ki lonje zouti yo ba li.

Doktè a pa te sispan ri li di mwen "Mwen pa kab kwè ke ou fè sa" lè ke mwen lonje twous zouti a ba li. Sa se dènye kalite travay scut. Ou pa te oblije fè sa. Yo rele travay scut tout kalite travay ke yon doktè oblije fè nan yon lopital. An règ jeneral yo pa bay etidyan doktè yo twòp travay scut pou ke yo kab gen tan fè sa ki pi enpòtan ki se aprann metye doktè a. "Mwen menm rele zanmi mwen nan New York e mwen di yo sa ke ou ap fè"

"Gen yon moun ki ta dwe pou fè travay sa" mwen reponn pandan ke mwen te ap ri" Mwen te gen lapenn pou li. Se yon sitiyasyon ki vreman dwòl" Mwen te admèt ke mwen te kontan pou mwen bay yon lòt moun pran responsabilite ede malad la pou yon ti moman. Nou konnen ke se pou jenn gason a te bay jèm la an maten sa a paske yo ta pral kòmanse tretman a nan apremidi a.

Vè pita ekip ematoloji onkoloji a te ap rankontre nan yon ti sal konferans kote ke yo te ap diskite ka tout patyan nan sèvis la, lè ke yon enfimyè parèt tèt li epi li di "viktwa. Li fè li" Nan doktè ki te nan sal la yon pati te anvi rele viv lòt yo te gen yon santiman soulajman. Enfimyè a ki te ap souri te ajoute ke: "Depatman iroloji a mande eske yo kapab kenbe twous zouti a,"

"Non Janmen" doktè ki responsab sal la te reponn "Eske ou pran li back, nou pral sèvi ak li pou malad pedyatri ki bezwen mete jèm yo nan labank."

"Natirèlman" enfimyè a di ak tout konfyans nan tèt li "Yo kapab fè twous zouti pa yo."

Sa ki motive moun ki antre nan branch laswenyaj pa sèlman doktè yo men tou lòt travayè ki ap okipe moun malad se chans yo genyen pou pote kontribisyon yo nan lavi yon kretyen vivan menm se ke pou trete yon maladi oswa rann la vi moun nan pi fasil. Men vle kwè ke ekip ki te ap travay ak patyan sa a (doktè yo, enfimyè yo travayè sosyal la, epi mwen menm etidyan a) nou ale pi lwen ke maladi a, nou trete yon moun. Kwake patyan nou a ki gen disètan ap swete joukkounye a ke li te antre tout antye nan vant latè, yon jou lè ke li geri ak kansè a li ap kab sèvi ak sa nou te sye fè pou li a pou li komanse lafanmi li. ☀

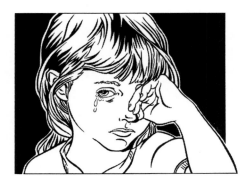

A Pool of Tears

By Samantha E. Feanny

Bang. Silence. A thousand tears.

As Gianni Versace lay lifeless on the front steps of his Miami Beach home, I sat on the Spanish Steps in Rome watching a fashion show come together. It was July 15, 1997, and I was 12 years old. I knew nothing of fashion, but I knew the name Versace.

Sitting and watching the flurry of excitement on the Steps was a well needed break from our busy tourist schedule of pointing and clicking at anything that looked remotely historical. As I gazed at models wearing beaded ball gowns in the sweltering midday Italian heat, something out of place caught my eye. A woman, no less beautiful than Aphrodite herself, looked as though she were in excruciating pain as she held a cell phone to her ear. She was dressed in white and her legs seemed impossibly long. When she put down the phone, she suddenly let out a piercing wail, "Perché Dio? Perché Gianni?" At that moment, everything stopped.

Thirteen years later, while working at the Miami-Dade County Health Department an unusual assignment captured my attention. A swimming pool inspection was going to take place at the old Versace mansion, Casa Casuarina. My colleague, Tracie, was assigned to go with the inspector, but this was by far the most exciting opportunity that popped up since I began working. With a bribe of a free lunch and a promise to keep my mouth shut, I weaseled my way onto the trip.

Three of us went on two pool inspections that day. The first was at a swanky South Beach hotel, where we simply flashed our badges and were given free reign to roam. When we arrived at Casa Casuarina, however, the scene was starkly different. Gianni Versace was South Beach royalty and we were mere peasants begging at the gate.

Despite the fact we were acting as the State and thus entitled to enter the property, which was now a posh hotel, we waited patiently in the sun. To stop the intense glare, Tracie pulled her sunglasses out of her bag and placed them on her face. Shining on her temple sat the iconic Medusa logo. I turned to her and said with a smile, "How fitting." As the temperature climbed to 100 degrees and a musty sea breeze went by, my mind wondered back to that day in Rome.

On the morning Gianni died, Donatella, his sister, had been busily preparing for the Fall Fashion Show on the Spanish Steps. When she received the news that Gianni had become the fifth victim of Andrew Cunanan, a suicidal spree killer hiding out in Miami Beach, she was devastated. Her attempt to get out of Rome to see her brother sent the city into utter madness as paparazzi stormed the nearby Hotel De La Ville where she was staying. Aware of the increasing chaos, my family and I tried to get out of the area, but were somehow swept up and into the crowd. We spent the rest of the day fighting for taxis and battling our way back to our hotel.

Standing outside Casa Casuarina's black and gold metal gate was different. I was dying to be a part of the Versace crowd this time. Perhaps the wait made it even more enticing, somewhat like being on the other side of the velvet rope at the hottest nightclub. I had walked by the mansion a hundred times, always pausing in front and wondering if I might be in the spot where Versace was gunned down on his doorstep. This time I would go inside.

Once the security guards and the maintenance crew confirmed our identity, the gate was opened. With Nick, our inspector, leading the way, we entered the courtyard. My eyes dashed back and forth at all the dazzling sights. It was as though we had walked into an issue of Italian Vogue. There were statues of bronze mermaids, lounge chairs covered in the finest of tapestries, grass that looked too good to walk on, hand-painted frescoes on every wall, and a marble mosaic floor patterned in the Versace logo – the head of Medusa. Then we saw the pool.

For a second I think we all forgot our reason for visiting the mansion. We actually had a job to do other than gawking. However, this was a pool so stunning that Michelangelo would have taken a second look. As we approached, Hector, the head of maintenance, smirked, "Nice, huh?" There were many words I could have used to describe that pool. Plain old "nice" was not one of them.

The pool, shaped like a half moon with two extended wings, is framed by marble tile and lays against the South wall. The wall, covered in frescoes, reminded me of Renaissance era cathedrals. However, the real glamour came from under the water.

The sunlight that escaped through the palms surrounding the property glistened curiously on the surface of the water. Sparks of every color splashed off the wall onto the two large marble mermaid vases at the corners of the pool. I approached the edge of the water, looked down, and saw the reason this pool seemed so magical. Every inch of the pool floor was covered in hand-laid mosaic tiles, no bigger than a square inch. There were yellow tiles, red tiles, green, orange, and a blue that could easily have been crafted from lapis lazuli. The shiniest and most striking tiles, however, were the gold ones. In the center of the pool, the tiles once again formed the image of Medusa with her snake-like hair and whose piercing eyes seemed to follow our every move.

It is hard to picture this house being the site of such grief. It was even harder to know that we were there to deliver more heartache. The same tile that had transfixed my gaze posed a risk to the guests of the hotel. Nick had explained this to me earlier, "If someone were to fall in and start drowning the tile would obstruct a possible rescuer's view." I thought of Narcissus staring at his reflection, and then imagined some tourist falling into the pool after meeting Medusa's gaze. Rules were rules and this pool violated so many of them.

Nick and Tracie broke the bad news, "the pool has to be closed... guests can drown...too much tile...no depth markings...slippery surface." As Hector took this all in, the three of us stood there with utter guilt on our faces. Versace may have rolled just a touch in his grave.

Not knowing what else to do, we began walking towards the entrance. I could see it in everyone's eyes, we did not want this to be the end of our Versace mansion story.

Just as we were a few feet from the metal gate, Tracie suddenly piped up, "Maybe there is something else we can do." Everyone stopped and turned to her. She looked at Hector and asked, "Do guests really use the pool much?"

"I haven't seen anybody in it," Hector responded.

"Then why keep it as a pool? What if you left it as is, and instead of using it as a pool, why not make it a fountain?" As Tracie finished her sentence, I could see everyone's eyes light up.

We left that afternoon knowing no matter what, we would find a solution. Gianni Versace and Casa Casuarina were too much a part of Miami Beach for us to treat this as any other pool. Although Cunanan, much like Medusa in the tales of the ancient Greek, had left Versace frozen in time like a statue on his front door steps, we could not let another bit of his legacy crumble apart.

Samantha Feanny is a graduate of University of Miami School of Law and New York University. She presently works for the Miami-Dade County Health Department, Contracts Division. She is a native of Jamaica and a cat fancier.

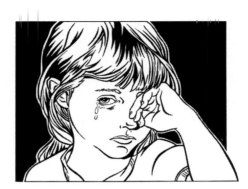

Una Piscina De Lagrimas

Por Samantha Feanny
Traducido por Ninfa Urdaneta

Bang. Silencio. Mil lágrimas.

Mientras Gianni Versace se encuentra sin vida en los escalones del frente de su casa en Miami Beach, yo me sentaba en las escalinatas españolas en Roma, mirando el desfile de moda que se llevaba a cabo. Era el 15 de Julio de 1997, y yo tenía 12 años. No sabía nada sobre la moda, pero conocía el nombre Versace.

Sentarse a mirar la exuberancia de la excitación sobre las escaleras era un receso bien necesitado en nuestro tan ocupado itinerario de visitar todo lo que pareciera remotamente histórico. Mientras yo daba una mirada a las modelos mostrando sus bordados vestidos de gala durante el sofocante calor del mediodía italiano, algo fuera de lugar me llamó la atención. Una mujer, no menos bella que la misma Afrodita, se veía como si estuviera experimentando un dolor insoportable mientras tenía el celular puesto en su oreja. Ella estaba vestida de blanco y sus piernas parecían imposiblemente largas. Cuando colgó el teléfono, ella inmediatamente dio un desgarrador gemido, "¿Perché Dio? ¿Perché Gianni?" En ese momento, todo paró.

Trece años después, mientras trabajaba para el Departamento

de Salud del Condado de Miami-Dade, una inusual tarea capturó mi atención. Una inspección de piscina iba a tomar lugar en la vieja mansión de Versace, Casa Casuarina. Mi colega, Tracie, fue asignada a ir con el inspector, pero esta era sobradamente la oportunidad más excitante que había surgido desde que comencé a trabajar. Con un soborno de almuerzo gratis y la promesa de mantener mi boca cerrada, yo me colé en el viaje.

Tres de nosotros nos fuimos a inspeccionar piscinas ese día. La primera era en un ostentoso hotel de South Beach, en donde simplemente mostramos nuestras insignias y nos fue dado libre reino para merodear por todo el lugar. Cuando llegamos a Casa Casuarina, sin embargo, la escena era marcadamente diferente. Gianni Versace era de la realeza de South Beach y nosotros éramos meros plebeyos rogando en la entrada.

A pesar del hecho que estábamos actuando en representación del Estado y así autorizados a entrar a la propiedad, la cual era ahora un elegante hotel, esperamos pacientemente bajo el sol. A fin de aminorar el intenso resplandor, Tracie sacó sus anteojos de sol de su cartera y se los puso en su cara. Brillando en su templo estaba el icónico logo de la Medusa. Me dirigí hacia ella y con una sonrisa le dije, "Cuan apropiado." Mientras la temperatura llegaba a 100 grados y una brisa húmeda soplaba, mi mente se trasladó tiempo atrás a ese día en Roma.

En la mañana que Gianni murió, Donatella, su hermana, se había estado preparando incesantemente para el Show de Moda de Otoño en las escalinatas españolas. Cuando ella recibió la noticia de que Gianni se había convertido en la quinta victima de Andrew Cunanan, un loco asesino suicida que se escondía en Miami Beach, ella estaba devastada. Su intento de salir de Roma para ver a su hermano envolvió a la ciudad en una total locura mientras los paparazzi rodeaban el cercano Hotel de la Ville donde ella se estaba hospedando. Concientes del creciente caos, mi familia y yo tratamos de salir del área, pero fuimos de cierta manera barridos hacia la multitud. Pasamos el resto del día peleando por taxis y batallando para regresar al hotel.

Estando fuera de la puerta de metal dorada y negra de Casa Casuarina era diferente. Me moría esta vez por ser parte de la multitud de Versace. Quizás el esperar lo hizo aún más atractivo, algo así como estar al otro lado del cordón de terciopelo a la entrada de la discoteca de moda. Yo he caminado por alrededor de la mansión cientos de veces, siempre pausando en frente de la misma, y siempre preguntándome si yo estaría en el sitio donde Versace fue asesinado en la puerta de su casa. Esta vez yo entraría.

Una vez que los guardias de seguridad y el equipo de mantenimiento verificaron nuestras identidades, la puerta de entrada fue abierta. Con Nick, nuestro inspector, guiando el camino, entramos al patio de la mansión. Mis ojos recorrieron de arriba a abajo todo los deslumbrantes lugares. Era como haber entrado a una emisión italiana de Vogue. Había estatuas de bronce de sirenas. Sillas de sala cubiertas con la más fina tapicería, grama que se veía demasiado bien para pisarla, frescos pintados a mano en todas las paredes, y un mosaico de mármol en el piso basado en el logo de Versace – la cabeza de la Medusa. Luego vimos la piscina.

Por un momento pensé que todos olvidamos nuestra razón de estar visitando la mansión. Nosotros verdaderamente teníamos un trabajo que hacer además de mirar boquiabiertos. Sin embargo, esta era una piscina que te dejaba tan anonadada que el mismo Miguel Ángel la habría mirado de nuevo. Mientras nos acercamos, Héctor, el supervisor de mantenimiento, se medio sonrió, y dijo, "¿Bien, huh?" Había muchas palabras que yo pudiera haber usado para describir esa piscina. El simple "bien" no era una de ellas.

La piscina, en forma de media luna con dos alas extendidas, está revestida en losas de mármol y se encuentra contra la pared sur. La pared cubierta en frescos, me recordó las catedrales de la época del Renacimiento. Sin embargo, el glamour real venía del fondo de la piscina.

La luz del sol que se escapaba a través de las palmas que rodean la propiedad brillaba curiosamente sobre la superficie del agua. Destellos de cada color se esparcían de la pared sobre los dos grandes jarrones de las sirenas de mármol en las esquinas de la piscina. Yo me acerqué a la orilla del agua, miramos hacia abajo, y nos dimos cuenta de la razón por la que esta piscina parecía tan mágica. Cada pulgada del piso de la piscina estaba cubierta por losas de mosaicos hechas a mano, no más grande que una pulgada cuadrada. Había losas amarillas, losas rojas, verdes, anaranjadas, y un azul que podía fácilmente haber sido hecho de lapislázuli. Sin embargo, las losas más brillantes y más sorprendentes eran las doradas. En el centro de la piscina, las losas otra vez formaban la imagen de la Medusa con su pelo en forma de culebras y cuyos ojos penetrantes parecían seguirnos en cada movimiento.

Es difícil imaginar que esta casa era el sitio de tan profunda pena. Era todavía más difícil saber que estábamos allí para dar más dolor. La misma losa que había petrificado mi mirada ponía un riesgo a los huéspedes del hotel. Nick me había explicado esto a mí con anterioridad, "Si alguien se cayera en la piscina y empezara a hundirse la losa podría obstruir la vista de un posible rescatador". Yo pensé en Narciso con su mirada fija en su reflección, y luego me imaginé a algún turista cayéndose adentro de la piscina después de encontrarse con la mirada petrificante de la Medusa. Las reglas son las reglas y esta piscina violaba muchas de ellas.

Nick y Tracie dieron las malas noticias, "la piscina debe ser cerrada…los huéspedes pueden ahogarse…demasiada losa…no hay señalización de profundidad…superficie resbalosa." Mientras Héctor explicaba todo esto, nosotros tres permanecíamos allí con una cara de extrema culpabilidad. Versace podía estar retorciéndose en su tumba.

Sin saber que más hacer, empezamos a caminar hacia la entrada. Yo podía verlo en la cara de todos, nosotros no queríamos que este fuera el final de nuestra historia de la mansión Versace.

Solo cuando estábamos a pocos pies de la puerta de metal, Tracie saltó diciendo, "Quizás haya algo que podamos hacer." Todos paramos y nos giramos hacia ella. Ella miró a Héctor y preguntó, "¿Los huéspedes en verdad utilizan mucho la piscina?"

"No he visto a nadie en ella," Héctor respondió.

"¿Entonces para qué mantenerla como piscina? ¿Que tal si tú la dejas como está, y en vez de utilizarla como piscina, por qué no hacerla una fuente?" Cuando Tracie finalizó su oración, pude ver que los ojos de todos nosotros se iluminaron.

Nos fuimos esa tarde sabiendo que de una forma u otra, encontraríamos una solución. Gianni Versace y Casa Casuarina eran una parte muy importante de Miami Beach para nosotros tratarla como cualquier otra piscina. A pesar de que Cunanan, similar a la Medusa en las historias de la antigua Grecia, dejaron a Versace congelado en el tiempo como una estatua en las escalinatas de su puerta de entrada, no podíamos dejar que otra parte de su legado se despedazara.

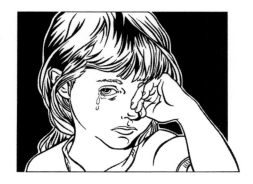

Yon pisin plen ak krye

Se Samantha E. Feanny ki ekri istwa sa a
Translation: Roland Pierre

Bang. Pa gen yon bwi. Mil gout dlo, krye.

Pandan ke Gianni Versace kouche rèd mò nan mach eskalye ki devan kay Miami Beach li a, mwen chita sou mach eskalye yon rele Spanish nan vil Rome ap gade yon defile mòd ki ap dewoule. Se te 15 juyè, 1997, e mwen te gen douzan. Mwen pa te konnen twòp bagay sou zafè la mòd men mwen te konnen non Versace a.

Pandan ke mwen te ap chita epi ke mwen te ap gade tout aktivite ki te blayi sou eskalye Spanish nan vil Rome la, se te yon ti repo ke nou te byen bezwen nan orè tourist nou a ki te plen twòp nan gade ak lonje dwèt sou tout sa ki te sanble ak istwa ansyen. Pandan ke nan mitan chalè anraje ki te genyen a midi nan peyi Itali, mwen te ap gade mannken ki te abiye ak rad bal ki te pèle, gen yon bagay ki pa te nan plas li ki te atire atansyon nou. Te gen yon fanm bèl tankou deès Aphrodite ki te sanble ke lit e gen yon doulè terib kit e ap ravaje kò li pandan ke li te kenbe yon telefòn selilè nan zorèy li.

Li te abiye ak yon rad blan epi janb li yo te parèt long anpil. Lè ke li depose telefòn la

Li pete yon rèl ki tap pèse zorèy moun li te rele:"Perché Dio? Perché Gianni?" Lè sa a tout aktivite te sispann.

Trèzan apre pandan ke mwen te ap travay nan Depatman Lasanté Miami-Dade County gen yon lòd pou ale fè yon travay ki te kapte atansyon mwen. Yon enspeksyon pisin ta pral fèt nan vye palè Versace, ki rele Casa Casuarina. Kolèg travay mwen Tracie te resewa lòd pou li ale ak yon enspektè, men se te pi bèl okasyon pou mwen te divèti mwen ki te genyen depi ke mwen te komanse ap travay nan Depatman Lasanté Miami-Dade la. Lè ke mwen soudwaye li ak pwomès pou mwen bali manje midi epi ke mwen te pwomèt li ke mwen pa tap pale ditou sou enspeksyon a mwen chikin kò mwen pou mwen ale nan enspeksyon a.

Nou touletwa te ale nan de enspeksyon pisin jou sa a. Premye a se te nan yon lotèl gran lix nan South Beach, kote ke nou te sèlman montre kat identifikasyon nou epi yo te banou dwa pou nou antre fè travay nou. Men lè ke nou te rive nan Casa Casuarina, se te yon lòt zafè paske Gianni Versace se te tankou wa nan South Beach epi ke nou se te tankou moun abitan ki travay latè ki te ap mande lacharite.

Malgre ke nou te nan travay ofisyèl pou leta Florida epi ke akòz de sa nou te gen dwa pou antre sou pwopriete a ki te tounen yon lotèl gran klas pou gwo zouzoune, nou te oblije rete ap tann nan solèy la ak tout patyans nou. Pou anpeche reflè solèy la nan je li, Tracie rale linèt solèy li sot nan valiz li epi li mete yo nan je li. Siyn ke tout moun konnen ki te make bagay Versace fè e ki se yon Medusa te ap klere sou bò tanp li.

Mwen vire gade li epi mwen di li pandan ke mwen te ap ri gade ki jan sa byen tonbe ak kote ke nou ye a. Kòm tanperati a te grenpe 100 degre epi te gen yon ti briz lanmè ki te soufle lide mwen vinn ale tounen sou jou sa a nan vil Rome la.

Jou maten ke Gianni te mouri a, sè li Donatella te okipe ap prepare pou defile mòd ki te fèt nan sezon otòn la sou eskalye Spanish nan vil Rome la. Lè ke li te resewa nouvèl ke Gianni te tounen senkyèm victim de Andrew Cunanan, yon moun ki te vle tiye tèt li epi tou ki te ap mache tiye moun ki te ap kache nan Miami Beach, sa te frape li anpil. Lè ke li te ap eseye soti nan Rome pou ale wè frè li sa te mete vil la nan yon eta foli ak tout paparazzi ki te kouvri zòn otou Hotel De La Ville kote ke li te desann. Lè ke fanmi mwen te wè tout tibilans san kontwòl, yo menm ak mwen te eseye kite vil la, men foul moun yo te pote nou ale. Nou pase rès jounen a ap goumen pou jwen yon taxi epi ap eseye jwen wout pou nou tounen nan lotèl kote ke nou te desann la.

Lè ke nou te kanpe devan baryè nwa et dore Casa Casuarina se te yon lòt bagay.

Fwa sa a mwen te ap mouri anvi pou mwen te pami foul ki te ap swiv Versace yo. Pètèt paske mwen te oblije tann tout tan sa a te fè ke mwen te pi enterese fwa sa a, se te tankou ke mwen te lòt bo kòd vlou nan pi bon nan bwat de nwi yo. Mwen te pase bòkote palè a san fwa, mwen te toujou kanpe devan li ap mande tèt mwen si kote ke mwen te ye a se te kote menm ke yo te tire Versace ak revolvè a sou mach peron kay li a. Fwa sa a mwen te kapab antre.

Yon fwa ke sekirite gad la ak ekip ki okipe antretyen pwopriete a te asire li ke nou se te moun nou di ke nou te ye yo, yo te louvri baryè a. Ak enspektè nou a ki te rele Nick ki te pran devan, nou antre nan lakou pwopriete a. Je mwen gade a dwat a gòch tout bèl kote ki te eblouyi moun ak jan yo te bèl. Se te tankou nou te ap mache nan yon nimewo revi yo rele Vogue la. Te gen estati lasirèn ki te fèt an bronz, te gen chèz pou salon ke te kouvri ak pi bèl tapisri, gazon ki te parèt two bèl pou moun mache sou li, penti sou plat fre yo rele fresco sou tout mi yo, epi atè a te gen yon mosayik ki te fèt ak mab ki te gen desen siyn Versace a ladan li- tèt Meduse la; Epi lè sa a nou wè pisin la.

Pandan yon segond mwen kwè ke nou tout te blye pou ki rezon ke nou te vinn vizite palè a. Nou te gen yon jòb pou nou te fè nou pa te vini pou nou rete egare bouch louvri.Men se te yon pisin tèlman eblouyisan ke menm atist Michelangelo tap rete pou li gade tou. Kòm nou te ap apwoche Hector ki se te chèf ekip antretyen a gade nou ak yon souri ki te ensolan «bèl bagay sòw di?" Te gen anpil mo mwen te ka sèvi pou di kijan ke pisin la te ye men bèl tou senpleman pa te yon ladan yo.

Pisin la te gen fòm yon mwatye lalin ak de zèl ki te sòti chak bò li, li te antoure ak karo mab epi li te apiye sou mi ki te nan sid pwoprietye a. Mi pisin la ki te kouvri ak tablo fèt ak plastè ke yo te pentire sa yo rele frescoes yo, te fèm sonje katedral ki te fèt nan epòk Renaissance la. Men bote pisin la se te nan pati ki te anba dlo a.

Solèy la te ap filtre nan mitan branch pye palmist yo ki te antoure pwopriete a te ap glise dwòlman sou sifas dlo a. Zèklè ki te tout koulè te gaye andeyò mi a sou de gwo potaflè ki te fèt ak mab e ki te gen fòm lasirèn ke yo te mete nan kwen pisin la. Mwen apwoche bò dlo a, mwen gade anba epi mwen wè poukisa pisin la te sanble ke li se te yon bagay majik. Tout pous a tè pisin la te kouvri ak karo mozaik ke yo te poze a la men, epi karo yo pa te pi gwo ke yon pous kare. Karo mozaik yo te jòn, yo te rouj, yo te vèt, oranj, epi yon ble ke yo ta kab kwè ki te taye nan pyè lapiz lazuli. Men Karo ki te pi piti e ki te pi frape atensyon moun plis yo se te sa ki te koulè lò yo.Nan mitan pisin la karo yo te fè potre yon Medusa ak cheve li ki te tankou sèpan epi je li li te ap fixe moun te sanble ke li te swiv tout mouvman ke ou te ap fè.

Li difisil pou yon moun imajine ke yon bagay tris konsa tankou sa ki te pase la te rive nan yon kote konsa. Li te pi tris toujou pou ke nou te konnen ke nou menm ta pral pote plis move nouvèl traka toujou. Men karo mozayik ki te eblouyi mwen a te yon danje pou moun ki te desann nan lotèl la. Nick te esplike mwen sa avan "Si yon moun ta tonbe nan pisin la epi li ta kòmanse nwaye karo mozayik yo te ap anpeche moun ki vinn sekouri li a wè" Lè sa a mwen te sonje Narcissus ki te ap gade tèt li n nan dlo a, epi mwen imajine kèk tourist ki tonbe nan pisin la apre ke je li kontre ak pa Medusa; La lwa se la lwa epi pisin la te an kontravansyon avèk twòp keksyon lalwa.

Nick and Tracie bay move nouvèl la " Se pou yo fèmen pisin la pou yo pa sèvi ak li...moun ki desann nan lotèl la kab nwaye ....twòp ti karo mozayik...yo pa te make pwofondè pisin la...sifas la twò glise."Kòm Hector te ap ankese tout sa ke nou te di li yo, nou tou le twa te kanpe la ak figi nou ki te montre ke nou te santi nou koupab anpil. Versace dwe woule enpe nan tonb li.

Nou pat konnen ki lòt bagay ke nou te ka fè kidonk nou kòmanse pran wout pou nou soti. Mwen te wè nan je nou tout ke nou pa ta kab kite istwa palè Versace a fini konsa.

Lè ke nou te prèske rive kèk pye lwen baryè metal la, Tracie di tou ba nan yon ti souf "Pètèt gen yon lòt bagay ke nou kab fè" Tout moun te sispan mache yo rete pou yo te vire gade li. Li gade Hector epi li mande li «eske klyan lotèl la konn sèvi ak pisin la anpil,"

"Mwen pa janm wè pèson ladan li" Hector te reponn.

"Alò pouki sa pou nou kenbe li kòm yon pisin? E si ou te kite li jan ke li ye epi olye de sèvi ak li kòm yon pisin pouki nou npa fè li tounen yon fontèn? Kòm Tracie te ap fini fraz li a mwen te wè je tou moun ki te ap briye.

Nou te vire ale jou apremidi sila a alòske nou te konnen ke kèlke swa jan a nou te ap jwen yon solisyon.Gianni Versace and Casa Casuarina se twòp yon pati nanm vil Miami Beach pou nou te trete enspeksyon sa tankou enspeksyon nenpòt ki kalite pisin. Menmsi asasen yo rele Cunanan menm jan ak Medusa nan fab ansyen Grèk yo, te kite Versace jele pou tout tan tankou yon estati sou mach pewon kay li a, nou pa ta kab kite yon lòt ti moso pati nan eritaj li kite a dekonstonbre.

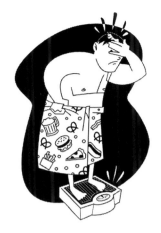

Fat Belly

By Mort Laitner

In the morning light, I stood naked in front of the mirror and screamed, "How did I let this happen?" Staring at my gut, my hands grasping the fat, I nodded in disbelief mouthing the words "What a catastrophe! Quelle horreur!"

I avoided studying my midsection for decades. Avoidance led to denial and denial led to extra large clothing. What I saw was not a pretty picture. Every year I let the inches grow. I refused to stand on scales, look in mirrors or do anything that would unmask my girth. In my head, I did not have a fat belly...A gordito, yes. But not a gordo. I watched "The Biggest Loser" but that was not me.

Friends gently voiced their disgust. "Mort, lose some pounds or you'll get sick...heart attack, diabetes, cancer."

Even my gutless surgeon, after fixing my hernia, spoke up about my dilemma. He sent a blunt message through my family, "Tell him to lose that fat!" He had a right to be angry because my girth got in the way of his surgery.

Covering my nakedness and shame with a towel plastered with pictures of pilsner, pretzels and pizza, I realized that today was weigh-in day at my weight loss center. It was time to strategize. I needed to drink decaf coffee to make sure I go to the bathroom. I must dress in my weigh-in uniform: short-sleeve shirt, shorts and sandals.

While shaving and watching the stubble wash down the drain, I remembered a high school wrestling buddy. He taught me to lighten up before a wrestling match. He'd say, "You're too close to your weight limit. Before you get on the ref's scale, shave off some of your body hair. You'll lose a few ounces."

As I drove, I felt the rush of heading toward the scale. This anticipatory ritual has become simultaneously fun and nerve-racking. Weight-loss success tastes sweeter than charoset... failure as bitter as maror.

Parking my car in the space furthest from the center, I enjoyed speed-walking every extra step.

Entering the center, I scanned two banners attached to the wall. The large one read, "Don't sit when you can stand; don't stand when you can walk; and don't walk when you can run." I wondered why the center had neglected to put a few stationary bikes in their waiting room. The smaller banner read, "Diets are temporary, lifestyle changes are forever."

I stood and reread three photo-testimonials splattered on the wall:

I wanted to feel like a new person;

My energy level went up and my blood pressure went down;

I never felt hungry.

These biggest loser photographs are segregated on walls of men, women, or loving couples (program partners). These lovers' eyes sent messages of adoration. They hold hands...their arms wrapped around each other. Weight loss has brought love back into their lives. The camera's lens captured their mutual sexual attraction.

I turned from the pictures and glanced around the waiting room: a fiftyish mom with her twentyish-year-old disabled daughter, a three-hundred pound young male drinking a super-sized soda, and two women who were maybe ten pounds over weight. A counselor entered and yelled, "Sue, so good to see you. How many pounds have you lost so far?"

Sue's mom replied, "Fifty –two." The room exploded in applause. The three-hundred pounder, who had not yet paid his initiation fee, was hooked. I rewarded the counselor with a "you-sly-devil" stare.

My name was called. I jumped to attention, headed to the scale, and stripped off my suspenders and glasses. I emptied my pockets of

Blackberry, wallet and keys. I patted myself down, like a cop frisking a derelict. I climbed, prayed and watched the numbers fly by my eyes. My counselor smiled, "Good job. You lost three pounds this week."

I sighed relief and answered, "Thanks for the encouragement, but I have miles to go before I reach my goal."

The next morning, standing in front of the mirror, I studied my naked contour. Rain clouds obscured the light entering the room and a tear welled in my eye as I asked my mirror, "Will I ever lose this fat belly?" ✺

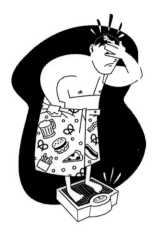

El Barrigón

Por Mort Laitner
Traducido Por Ninfa Urdaneta

A la luz del amanecer, me paré desnudo en frente del espejo y grité, "¿Cómo dejé que esto pasara?" Mirando fijamente a mi panza, mis manos agarrando la grasa, moví mi cabeza articulando las siguientes palabras "¡Qué catástrofe! Quelle horreur!"

Yo evité estudiar mi sección media por décadas. El evitarlo me llevó a la negación y la negación me condujo a ropa extra larga. Lo que yo veía no era un bonito retrato. Cada año dejé que las pulgadas aumentaran. Me rehúse a pararme sobre las básculas, mirarme en espejos, o cualquier cosa que desenmascarara mi voluminoso contorno. En mi cabeza, yo no tenía una barriga grande…Un gordito, sí. Pero no un gordo. Yo vi "The Biggest Loser" pero ese no era yo.

Los amigos con tacto expresaron su disgusto. "Mort, pierde algunas libras o te enfermarás…ataques de corazón, diabetes, cáncer."

Inclusive mi cobarde cirujano, después de arreglar mi hernia, dio su opinión sobre mi dilema. El envió un contundente mensaje a través de mi familia, "¡Díganle que pierda peso!" El tenía el derecho de estar bravo ya que mi voluminoso contorno estaba en la vía de su cirugía.

Cubriendo mi desnudez y pena con una toalla cubierta con dibujos de vasos de cerveza, pretzels y pizza, me di cuenta que hoy era día de ir a pesarse en mi centro de pérdida de peso. Era tiempo de tener una estrategia. Necesitaba tomarme un café descafeinado para asegurarme de poder ir al baño. Yo debía vestirme en mi uniforme de ir a pesarse: Camisa manga corta, shorts y sandalias.

Mientras me afeitaba y miraba la barba bajar por el drenaje, me recordé de un compañero de lucha libre del bachillerato, quien me enseñó a encender un cigarrillo antes de la lucha libre. El decía, "Estás bien cerca de tu límite de peso. Antes de que te montes en la báscula del árbitro, aféitate algo del pelo que cubre tu cuerpo. Perderás algunas onzas."

Mientras manejaba, sentí el apuro de dirigirme a la pesa. Este ritual anticipado se ha hecho simultáneamente divertido y angustioso. El éxito en la pérdida de peso sabe más dulce que la charoset... el fracaso tan amargo como el maror.

Estacionando mi carro en el puesto de estacionamiento más lejano del centro, me divertí mucho con la corre caminata cada paso extra.

Entrando al centro, le eché un vistazo a dos carteles pegados en la pared. El grande decía, "No te sientes cuando te puedes parar; no te pares cuando puedes caminar; y no camines cuando puedes correr." Me pregunté por qué el centro no se ocupó de poner bicicletas inmóviles en la sala de espera. El más pequeño decía, "Las dietas son temporales, los cambios de estilos de vida son permanentes."

Me paré y leí tres testimonios con fotografías esparcidas en la pared:
Me quería sentir como una nueva persona;
Mis niveles de energía subieron y mi presión arterial bajó;
Nunca me sentí hambrienta.

Estas fotografías de grandes perdedores están segregadas en paredes de hombres, mujeres, o parejas de enamorados (compañeros de programa). Estos ojos de enamorados enviaban mensajes de adoración. Ellos se agarran las manos...sus brazos abrazados alrededor de cada uno. La pérdida de peso ha traído el amor de regreso a sus vidas. Los lentes de las cámaras capturaron su mutua atracción sexual.

Giré mi cabeza y di un vistazo alrededor de la sala de espera: Una madre en sus cincuenta con su discapacitada hija en sus vientes, un joven de trescientas libras tomando una soda de tamaño súper grande, y dos mujeres que probablemente tenían diez libras de más. Un orientador entró y gritó, "Sue, que bueno verte. ¿Cuántas libras has perdido hasta ahora?"

La mamá de Sue replicó, "Cincuenta y dos." La sala se llenó de aplausos. El que pesaba trescientas libras, quien no había pagado su inscripción, fue agarrado. Yo recompensé al orientador con una mirada de expresión de cariño y admiración.

Mi nombre fue llamado. Puse atención de inmediato, me dirigí a la báscula, me quité los tirantes y anteojos. Vacíe mis bolsillos de Blacberry, billetera y llaves. Me pasé las manos por todo el cuerpo chequeándome como un policía revisa a un marginado. Yo me monté sobre la báscula, recé y miré los números con mi propios ojos. Mi orientador sonrío, "Buen trabajo. Perdiste tres onzas esta semana."

Divisé alivio y respondí, "Gracias por tu alentamiento, pero tengo millas que recorrer antes de alcanzar mi meta."

La siguiente mañana parándome en frente de mi espejo, estudié mi desnudo contorno. Nubes de lluvia obscurecieron la luz que entraba al cuarto y una lágrima llenó mi ojo mientras yo le preguntaba a mi espejo, "¿Alguna vez yo rebajaré este barrigón?" ✺

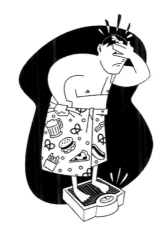

Gwo Vant

By Mort Laitner
Translation Roland Pierre

Anba limyè youn ti solèy maten ki fèk ap parèt, mwen kanpe devan youn miwa epi m pantan kifè m rele anmwe, " Kijan m fè kite sa rive?" Mwen fè youn kout je sou fal mwen, etan m ap leve pil grès vant mwen ak men m. Mwen souke tèt mwen kòmsi mwen paka konprann pandan mwen ap di tèt mwen " Ki katastwòf sa a! Ala de koze!"

Mwen te toujou kabre ekzamine vant mwen pandan anpil rekòlt kafe. Sa je pa wè, kè pa tounen ki al fòse mwen achte pi gwo rad pou m met sou mwen. Sa m te wè a vi n pa bèl ditou. Ane vini, ane ale se pa mele m sa, M ap manje m ap gwosi. Mwen refize pran pwa mwen, gade lan youn miwa se pa pale, osinon fè nenpòt lòt bagay ki ap fè m dekouvri lajè m te gentan rive. Lan tèt mwen, se pa avèk mwen wap pale, ki vant... patat, epi. Mwen ka pata, mwen mwen pa patatsi. Mwen gade film yo rele " Nèg ki pi pèdan" an angle "The Biggest Looser", se pa avèk mwen w ap pale.

Zanmi ap banm ti tèk detanzawot pou montre ke yo konsène." Mort, kilè w ap pedi enpe lan grès ki sou lestomak w a anvan li fè w règleman...fè kè w rete, ba w dyabèt sikre, e menm kansè pou touye w."

Menm ti chèchkobanza yo bay pou doktè m lan, ki te ede m anpil lè mwen te manke kokobe lan leve pwa ki twò lou pou mwen, te mete m chita pou li detaye pwoblèm sa ka ban mwen. Li te menm voye youn komisyon bay fanmi mwen, "Di l pou l pedi vye grès lap pote a!"Li te gen rezon fè m youn ti malelve denye fwa a, paske gwosè m te bal difikilte lè li te ap opere m.

Etan m byen vlope kò m ak tout wont mwen lan yon sèvyèt ki gen, alewè, youn pil foto byè, pen kòde, ak pidza sou li, mwen reyalize ke jodi a se jou pou m al pran pwa kò m lan sant de sante pou finalman mwen fè youn bagay ak sa. Lè a kouri vi n bout pou m planifye. Yo te ekzije nou bwè kafe san kafeyi'n ladan li pou mwen te ka al lan twolèt. Mwen te oblije mete rad leje si an ka, tankou chemiz manch kout, bout pantaloon ak youn zèl sapat lan pye m.

 Etan m ap gade bab mwen ki ap desann lan tou basen an padan kem ap raze, mwen sonje youn zanmi ki te bon patnè m lan match lit klas segondè. Li te di m pou m mete dlo lan divenm anvan mwen al lite ak pèsonn. Li te konn di m "Ou kòmanse rive pi gwo limit pwa kò w. Anvan w monte balans entrenè a, raze enpe pwal sou kò w. W ap pèdi o men de zons sou pwa kò w.

Etan m ap kondwi, mwen santi w sèl vètij. Randevou pou al monte balans sa a, vi n youn sèl zo ki pendye lan gòj mwen. Mwen vi n pa konn kote m met kò m. Afè pèdi pwa sa vi n tounen yon mòn kalvè ki dous tankou siwo si m reyisi…epitou anmè tankou lalwa si m ta bwè pwa.

Mwen egare machi n lan byen lwen pou m pran yon plezi mache vit anvan mwen rive lan sant lan, atansyon pa kapon.

Etan m fè sa pou m rantre, mwen voye je m sou mi moun yo. Mwen wè youn dividal ak youn pakèt pannkat kole sou li. Pi gwo a di" Pa chita lè w ka kanpe; pa kanpe lè w ka mache; epitou pa mache lè w ka kouri." Hey! Alò mwen mande tèt mwen, atò, pou ki rezon yo pat mete de twa bisiklèt lan rantre a pou moun amize yo si yo te kanpe sou kichòy? Alòs, lan mal lan mal nèt.

Etan m kanpe, mwen ap li twa rapò ak tout foto moun ki te pase lan pwogram layite sou mi a ki di:
    Mwen vle santi m youn lòt jan;
    Enèji mwen pran vòl monte lan syèl etan presyon m fè bèk atè.
    Mwen santi w sèl grangou pranm.

Sou youn arebò mi a, yo enstale tout moun ki te pèdi pwa avèk èd sant lan. Ou wè foto gason, fanm ak tout koup amourèz ki te vi n ansanm pou youn te sipòte lòt.

Zye amourèz yo lan foto a montre kijan youn te adore lòt. Lamen dan lamen... ou ta di se marasa. Afè pèdi pwa sa a fè yo vi n tounen out a di kòkòt ak figawo. Kamera a montre jan youn ta dechire lòt tèlman yo damou.

Pandan m bay foto yo do mwen pou m voye youn kout je sou sal pou moun tann lan: mwen wè youn ti granmoun ki gen apeprè sakan rekòlt kafe sou bwa tèt li, akonpanye de pitit fi li, ki pat fi n twò kòrèk pou m pa di kokobe, ki sanble ke l te genyen youn ventèn dane, ak youn jenn ti gason ki peze omwen twasan liv ki ap degiste youn michan gode kola, epi tou de lòt fanm kit e petèt bezwen pedi di liv. Youn lan konseye yo rantre lan sal la epi byen fò li di" Sue, sa fè youn grap plezi pou mwen wè w. Bon, di m non, konbyen liv w pèdi?"

Manman Sue pa menm kite l gen tan pou l reponn di" Senkant liv" Sa w tande a, sal la kraze ap bat bravo pou fè òlòj. Ti gason twa san liv la, ki potko men peye enskriyon an, pran la twa wa. Li manke dechire konseye a ak youn kout je.

Toudenkou, yo site non m. M leve kanpe, m mache sou balans lan, m retire bretèl mwen sou mwen ak tout linèt mwen. M retire tout sa m te gen lan pòch mwen, telefòn selilablakbèri, bous ak tout kle m. Mwen fouye tèt mwen toujou, ou ta di youn chèf k ap fouye yon vòlè. Mwen monte balans lan, m ap rele Bon Dye lan kè m etan m ap voye je sou nimewo yo k ap vole mounte. Konseye m lan souri, epi li di m "Mèkopliman. Ou pèdi twa liv semen sa a."

Kè m manke sòt lan bouch mwen, epi mwen di li " Mèsi deske w te ankouraje mwen, men mwen gen you bèl mòn pou m monte anvan m rive kote m ta sipoze ye a."

Lan demen maten, etan m kanpe jan manman m te fè m devan glas la, mwen ap adore fòm kò m. Nwaj lapli anpeche ti limyè solèy la rantre lan chanm lan, dlo sòti lan zye mwen etan m ap mande tè mwen " Eske m ap janm pedi vant sa a?" ✵

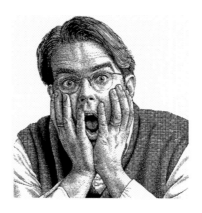

Head Games

By Mort Laitner

Surrounded by her friends and family, the FSU graduate cut into her celebratory cake. She parted the icing between Osceola's spear and Renegade's head. In an act of defiance, the cake knife bounced back. The graduate's face froze in disbelief. Her smile flipped into a grimace. She realized that her Seminole cake's top layer consisted of foam. The foam had been dressed in icing. The cake's purchaser hurriedly assisted her daughter in the removal of this faux layer. With all the anger of a child, embarrassed by a well-meaning parent, the graduate scraped the frosting from the foam layer. She then flung the icing onto the empty space left on her cake. This catapulting of garnet and gold helped burn away the negativity housed in her gut.

As my stomach hungered for the cake, I counted the witnesses, including the graduate. There were twenty. I watched seventeen of them eat cake. For the first time in my life, I was one of the three who neglected to partake. In my gut, I realized I had switched sides. I joined the smaller sized foam group.

My hungry eyes sent a short message to my brain. Oh my G-d. He has switched sides!

My stomach sent an SOS distress signal… "Feed me. Feed me. Feed me. A traitor is on board. Kill the traitor!"

My brain responded, "We'll teach this renegade a lesson he won't forget. There will be a high price for this insubordination. Does this sucker think he is in control?"

Pride lit up my face... change happens. I observed, collected data and abstained. I watched my fellow non cake eaters as they glowed in my eyes. They belonged on my team, on my tribe, by my side. Our team named the "losers" versus our worthy opponents the "gainers."

My resolve was again tested the next night surrounded by friends in a Thai restaurant our waitress served us bowls of rice. I usually ate one to two bowls. This time I abstained. I watched as my three compadres ate anywhere from one quarter to a half of a bowl of rice.

My inner voice screeches louder than my whimpering stomach, "How many calories in that starchy mountain of rice? I bet 700. One pound of fat equals 3500 calories." You're over your daily allotment of 1500 calories. Inner voice continued the rant, "Where is your calorie calculator? Do you want to be stranded on that weight loss plateau? Drink that glass of water with the lemon swimming in it. You have got to trick that stomach of yours."

My fork does not break the surface area of the mound. My hands pushed my bowl to the center of the table. The rice smelled like poison. I observed the rice eaters. They could not believe their eyes. Their inner voices whispered, "Maybe I ate too much rice. He beat me this time. It won't happen again." As they discretely glanced at my gut, they wondered if it had shrunk. I felt the euphoric joy of metabolized fats breaking down.

As I left the table, I chanted my new mantra, "Change your lifestyle, change your lifestyle, change your lifestyle."

I've lost eight and a half pounds in three weeks thanks to the diet program, liberal amounts of discipline sprinkled on my food and a number of head games. ☼

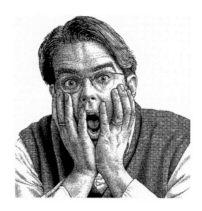

Juegos Mentales

Por Mort Laitner
Traducido por Frank Menendez y Francisco Menendez

Rodeada de sus amigos y familiares, la recién graduada de FSU cortaba el pastel de su fiesta. Ella separo el glasiado entre la lanza de Osceola y la cabeza del renegado. En un acto de desafío, el cuchillo de cortar el pastel rebotó. La cara de la posgrada se congeló de incredulidad. Su sonrisa se convirtió en una mueca. Se dio cuenta de que la capa superior de su pastel de Seminole consistía en espuma. La espuma se había vestido con el glasiado. El comprador de la torta rápidamente asistió a su hija a remover la capa imitadora. Con toda la ira de una niña, avergonzada por las buenas intenciones de su padre, la graduada raspó la espuda de la torta arrojándola hacia el espacio vacío que quedaba izquierda del pastel. Esta catapulta de granate y oro ayudó a quemar la negatividad alojada en el intestine de ella.

A medida que mi deseo de probar la torta crecía, conté los testigos, incluyendo a la postgrada. Habían veinte. Diecisiete de ellos se comieron el pastel. Por primera vez en mi vida, yo era uno de los tres que no tomé parte en eso. En mis entrañas, me dí cuenta que había cambiado de equipo. Me uní al grupo que selecionaba la espuma de menor tamaño.

Mis ojos hambrientos enviaron un corto mensaje a mi cerebro. !Oh Dios mio. Ha cambiado de equipo!

Mi estómago envío una señal de socorro... "Dáme de comer. Dáme de comer. Dáme de comer. Un traidor está a bordo. Maten al traidor! "Mi cerebro respondió: "Vamos a enseñarle a este renegado una lección que no olvidará. Habrá un alto precio por esta insubordinación. ¿Este tonto se cree que tiene el control?"

El orgullo iluminó mi rostro ... el cambio existe. He observado, he collecionado datos y pude abstenerme. Mis ojos se illuminaron al ver que mis compañeros no comían la torta. Pertenecían a mi equipo, a mi tribu, estaban a mi lado. Nuestro equipo, llamado los "perdedores," contra nuestros rivales los "ganadores."

Mi determinación fue probada de nuevo la noche siguiente, rodeado de amigos en un restaurante tailandés nuestra camarera nos sirvió platos de arroz. Por lo general yo comía de una a dos tazas. Esta vez me abstuve. Ví cómo mis tres compañeros comían de un cuarto a medio plato de arroz.

Los gritos de mi voz interna eran más fuerte que el quejido de mi estómago: "¿Cuántas calorías en esa montaña de almidón de arroz? Apuesto a que son 700. Una libra de grasa equivale a 3500 calorías. "Sobrepasastes tu dosis diaria de 1500 calorías. Mi voz interna continuó la diatriba, ¿Dónde está tu calculadora de calorías? ¿Quieres quedarte en este nivel? Bebe tu vaso de agua con el limón nadando en ella. Tienes que engañar a tu estómago."

El tenedor no rompió la superficie del montículo. Mis manos empujaron la taza al centro de la mesa. El arroz olía a veneno. Observé a los comedores de arroz. No podían creer lo que veían. Sus voces internas susurraban: "Tal vez comí demasiado arroz. Me ganó en esta ocasión. No volverá a suceder. "A medida que discretamente echaron un vistazo a mi estómago, se preguntaban si se había reducido. Sentí la alegría eufórica de que las grasas metabolizadas se rompían.

Al levantarme de la mesa, canté mi nueva canción, "Cambia tu estilo de vida, cambia tu estilo de vida, cambia tu estilo de vida..."

He perdido ocho libras y media en tres semanas gracias al programa de dieta, una cantidad abundante de disciplina salpicada en mi comida, y una serie de juegos mentales. !Que bien de mi parte!

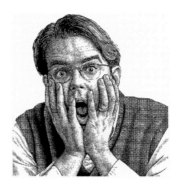

Jwèt ak tèt mwen

Se Mort Laitner ki ekri istwa sa a.
Translation: Roland Pierre

Etidyan ki fèk diplome nan inivèsite FSU gen zanmi ak fanmi li ki bòkote li lè ke li ap koupe gato pou fete okazyon remiz diplòm li. Li koupe glas gato a ant lans Osceola ak tèt Renegade la. Kouto pou gato a ap fè movèz fwa li pa koupe gato a epi li tounen vinn jwen li.Figi moun ki ap diplome a jele tankou glas tèlman ke li pa vle kwè sa ki ap pase a. Souri ki sou bouch li a tounen yon grimas. Lè sa a li realize ke premye etaj gato Seminole la se yon eponj.Yo degize eponj la ak glas pou glase gato . Moun ki te achte gato a kouri al ede pitit fi li pou li retire etaj gato ki fèt ak eponj la.Tankou yon ti moun ki kontrarye ki jennen devan paran li ki te gen bon entansyon, fi ki ap diplome a retire glas pou gato a sou eponj la. Epi lè sa a li li voye glas pou gato a sou sou espas vid ki rete sou dezyèm etaj ki se vre gato a. Lè ke li voye tout glas koulè rouj fonse ak koulè lò a sou vre gato a li li mete deyò tout move san ki te ap trakase li yo.

Pandan ke vant mwen ki vle manje gato a ap kòde ak grangou, mwen ap konte temwen yo, fi ki ap diplôme ladan temwen yo tou. Gen ven moun. Mwen gade pandan ke disèt ladan yo ap manje gato.Pou premye fwa nan lavi mwen, mwen se yonn nan twa moun ki pap manje nan gato ki ap separe a. Nan lide mwen mwen rann mwen kont ke mwen te chanje kan, mwen te al jwen ti gwoup moun ki pa te nan manje gato a.Je mwen ki te grangou voye yon mesaj bay sèvo mwen; O bondye li chanje kan. Vant mwen voye yon siyal pou mande osekou li di banm manje.Ban manje.Ban manje. Gen yon trèt ki an dedan ou.Tiye trèt la.

Sèvo mwen reponn nap bay vagabon sa a yon leson ke li pap janm bliye. Lap peye yon gwo pri paske li pa te soumèt li. Eske malen sa a kwè ke se li ki ap mennen?

Figi mwen te gen limyè sou li tèlman mwen te fyè de tèt mwen. Moun konn chanje. Mwen te gade, mwen te etidye sa ki te ap pase a, mwen te ranmase enfòmasyon epi mwen pa te manje gato.Mwen te ap gade moun ki tankou mwen pa te manje gato a, yo te parèt bèl plen ak limyè nan je mwen.Yo nan menm ekip ak mwen, yo nan tribi mwen a yo nan kan mwen. Ekip nou a rele moun ki ap pèdi yo ki kanpe anfas ak opozisyon djanm ke yo rele moun ki ap genyen yo.

Rezolisyon mwen mwen te anba kannon lòt swa a lè ke mwen te nan yon restoran Thai ak zanmi mwen epi ke moun ki ap sèvi manje a te ap sèvi bòl diri.Mwen abitye konn manje yon oswa de bòl diri. Fwa sa a mwen derefize diri mwen di non mèsi. Mwen te chita ap gade lè ke twa monkonpè mwen yo te manje yon ka epi menm mwatye yon bòl diri:

Vwa ki te nan tèt mwen a rele pi fò ke vant mwen ki te ap ple-nyen. Ki kantite kalori ki genyen nan mòn diri sa a? Mwen parye ke se 700.Yon liv grès egal 3500 kalori. Ou depase 1500 kalori ke ou gen pèmisyon pou ou manje chak jou a. Vwa ki nan tèt mwen a kontinye ap fè mwen repròch "Kote bagay pou ou kalkile ki kantite kalori ke ou ap pran nan manje chak jou? Eske ou vle ret kole ak menm pwa ki derefize desann la? Bwè vè dlo ak sitron ki ap naje ladan li a. Se pou ou trompe vant ou."

Fouchèt mwen pa antre nan mòn diri ki nan bòl la. Men mwen pouse bòl diri a lwen nan mitan tab la.Diri sila a santi tankou pwa-zon. Mwen ap fixe moun ki ap manje diri yo. Yo pa vle kwè sa ke yo wè ak je yo a. Vwa ki nan tèt yo ap di "pètèt nou te manje twop diri. Li kale nou fwa sa a. Sa pap rive ankò." Pandan ke yo ap gade mwen anba je pou mwen pa remake ke yo te ap gade mwen.Yo mande tèt yo eske gwosè mwen fè yo ti bese. Lè sa a mwen santi kè kontan ke mwen genyen akòz de grès ki te ap fonn nan kò mwen.

Pandan ke mwen te ap leve sòt sou tab la mwen chante nouvo re-fren mwen a "Chanje jan ke ou ap viv, chanje jan ke ou ap viv, chanje jan ke ou ap viv."

Mwen pèdi yit liv edmi nan twa semen granmèsi yon pwogram dayèt, anpil disiplin mwen soupoudre sou manje mwen, epi kèk jwèt ke mwen fè ak tèt mwen.

How to Contact the Editors
Call for Submissions
Order Additional Copies

Healthy Stories welcomes letters, stories, poems and recipes from its readers. Please e-mail to HealthyStories.net or mail to:

Healthy Stories
Editorial Board
8323 NW 12th Street
Suite 214
Miami, Florida 33126

Book Prize

Healthy Stories proudly announces the Healthy Stories Book Prize. All authors or poets must submit their health related short stories, poems or recipes by February 1, 2012. Winners will be published and receive three copies of Healthy Stories. No reading fee. Notification by March 1, 2012.

About the Editors

MORT LAITNER

Mort Laitner has practiced law for 36 years. He commenced practicing family law with the Legal Aid Society of Baton Rouge, Louisiana. His next job was with Legal Services of Greater Miami where his unit handled approximately 600 cases a year.

Since 1977, he has been the chief legal counsel for the Miami-Dade County Health Department, where he specializes in public health law.

Mort has taught at Barry University, University of Miami, School of Medicine, St. Thomas University, and Miami-Dade College. He has lectured throughout Florida and Georgia on public health issues.

He has handled high-profile cases which received coverage on the CBS Nightly News, Life Magazine, Money Magazine and the New York Times.

He is the author or co-author of eleven books, including:

Quarantine Preparing for the Attack Small Pox: Field Exercises, A how to Manual for a Beginner's Level Field Exercises

SARS: A Quarantine and Isolation Manual for Severe Acute Respiratory Syndrome

It is Just a Matter of Time, Recommendations that can Save Your Life

Healthy Stories 2007 - 2012

How to Create a Public Health Film Festival

He has produced and directed Pandemic, an avian influenza film. He has also co-chaired the Mango Writer's Conference.

Mort lives with his wife, Shelley, and has raised three sons, Jason, Travis, and Blake.

HEATHER BEATON

Heather L. Beaton was born in Miami, Florida. After graduating from Florida State University in 1999 with a degree in Political Science, Heather attended the University of Florida, Levin College of Law. She graduated with her Juris Doctorate in May 2002 with honors. Heather is a member of the Florida Bar. She currently practices law at the Miami-Dade County Health Department in the areas of contract, administrative and labor law. Heather lives with her husband, Marcos, their daughter, Kaitlyn, son Allan and a very large Boston Terrier, Blackjack.

TRACIE L. DICKERSON

Tracie L. Dickerson was born in Galveston, Texas. Tracie received her Bachelor of Science in Maritime Administration from Texas A & M University, her Juris Doctor from University of Miami's School of Law, a Masters in Public Health and an Environmental Health Certificate from Florida International University. She is currently pursuing her Ph.D. in Environmental Public Health. Tracie is a senior attorney for the Miami-Dade County Health Department, specializing in Environmental Health Law. She is a member of the Florida Bar, and a member of the U.S. District Courts for the Southern, Middle and Northern Districts of Florida and the Southern and Northern Districts of Texas. She has also published in the South Florida History Magazine.

Tracie is an active member of the Junior Leauge of Miami, Daughters of the American Revolution, the Order of the Eastern Star and the Florida International University Alumni Association. Tracie is recently engaged, and is looking forward to her upcoming wedding.

SAMANTHA FEANNY

Samantha E. Feanny was born in Kingston, Jamaica. She received her Bachelor of Arts in History from New York University in 2006 and her Juris Doctor from the University of Miami School of Law in 2009, both with honors. Samantha is a member of the Florida Bar and works as an attorney for the Miami-Dade County Health Department. She specializes in HIV/AIDS contracts and procurement law, and labor relations.

CAROLINE GLICK

Caroline A. Glick is a native of Miami Beach, Florida. She received her Bachelor of Arts in Communication Studies from the University of Minnesota in 2006, and her Juris Doctor from Nova Southeastern University in 2009, both with honors. Caroline is a member of the Florida Bar and works as an attorney for the Miami-Dade County Health Department.

SAM GONAS

Sam Gonas was born and raised in Coral Gables, Florida. He graduated high school from Culver Military Academy in Indiana and then went to Tucson, Arizona to receive his B.F.A. in Media Production at The University of Arizona in 1995. Sam is currently a Juris Doctor candidate at Florida International University College of Law with an expectation to sit for the Florida Bar Exam in February 2014.

Along with pursuing his J.D., Sam is a spring 2012 intern with the Miami-Dade County Health Department's legal division. Prior to law school, he practiced real estate in the Naples/Ft. Myers area and remains the broker/co-owner of American Diamond Real Estate, LLC in Naples, FL. When he used to have spare time, Sam enjoyed fishing for snook in Southwest Florida and taking in a football game or two.

LAUREN E. McGURK

Lauren E. McGurk is a native of Orlando, Florida. She received her Bachelor of Arts in History from the University of Florida in 2009, and is receiving her Juris Doctor from Florida International University in May 2012 with honors. In law school, Lauren has been especially active in environmental advocacy, particularly in Everglades Restoration.

FRANK MENENDEZ

Frank Menendez was born in Cuba and raised in Spain. He received his Bachelor of Arts in Education from Florida International University in 2004, and his Juris Doctor from the University of Miami School of Law in 2009. Frank is a member of the Florida Bar.

ROLAND PIERRE

Roland R. Pierre was born and raised in Petion-Ville, Haiti in 1963. In Haiti, he attended "Lycée Francais" and "Lycée de Petion-Ville" where he earned his Baccalaureate First & Second Part. While he was pursuing his Baccalaureate, he attended Jamaica School of Business and the Haitiano American Institute to learn Telecommunications (Telephones Switchboard) and practice his English. He moved to the US (Miami) in 1986. In 1995, he received his Associate of Science (AS), and ART (AA) degrees in Computer Information Systems Analysis (CISA), and Management Information Systems

(MIS) from Miami-Dade Community College. In 1999, he graduated from Florida International University with a degree of Bachelors of Sciences in Business Administration & Management Information Systems. In 2001, he earned his Masters of Science (MSMIS) degree from Florida International University with an overall GPA of 3.56. He enjoys reading technological periodicals, watching basketball, going to the gym, and playing soccer. He is a big FAN of sports specially basketball. He is always connected with the NBA and the local 790 The Ticket Sport Radio station. He is a member of Florida International University Alumni Association.

PHILIP E. REICHERT

Phil Reichert was born in Jacksonville, North Carolina to a New York dad who spent 26 years as a pilot in the US Marine Corps and a Tennessee mom who stayed home to raise three boys. Phil lived in several interesting places (mostly aboard military bases) that include Hawaii, Okinawa, California, Texas, Virginia, and, of course, Florida. He attended eleven schools between kindergarten and twelfth grade. Among Phil's passions are, writing (articles, a book, manuals and keeping a journal for over 38 years), music (listening and playing), art (observing and creating) and antique and classic automobiles (there's a 1957 Chevy in his garage awaiting restoration). Phil has a Bachelor's Degree in Communications from Florida State University and Masters Degree in Public Health from the University of South Florida. He has over 32 years in the public health sector working in sexually transmitted disease and HIV programs. He currently administers the statewide Hepatitis Prevention Program in Tallahassee. He and his wife Becky, raised three boys, Brandon, Benjamin and Adam.

J.D. SHINGLES

J.D. Shingles is originally from rural southwest Georgia. He moved to Miami in 1982 to work for the Grand Union Company, a grocery retailer, and Miami has since been his home. He received his Bachelor's degree in Business Administration, Management from the Fort Valley State University. He has volunteered at the Sant La Haitian Community center as an income tax preparer and has served as a Guardian Ad Litem. Mr. Shingles enjoys watching a good movie, mentoring, reading, fishing and traveling, whenever time permits. He is an active member of Theta Rho Sigma Chapter of the Phi Beta Sigma Fraternity, Incorporated.

AMY TEJIRIAN

Amy Tejirian is originally from Calgary, Alberta, Canada. She received her Bachelor of Arts degree with honors in Communication and French from the University of California at Santa Barbara. She continued her studies at the University of Miami School of Law where she received a Juris Doctorate. Amy is a member of both the Florida and California Bars. She is a member of the U.S. District Court for the Southern District of Florida. Amy has a Certificate of Public Health from the University of Florida and is pursuing a Master's in Public Health from the same institution. Amy was a kindergarten teacher for the Los Angeles Unified School District before she became an attorney. Amy has been in her current position as an attorney for the Miami-Dade County Health Department for over seven years. She speaks French and Armenian fluently. On her free time, she likes to go curling, go the beach and attend Florida Panthers games, although her favorite hockey team is the Calgary Flames.

NINFA URDANETA

Ninfa Urdaneta is an attorney licensed to practice in the state of Florida and Venezuela. Originally from Maracaibo, Venezuela, she moved to the United States when she got married, and has two adorable children. She received her Juris Doctor from Nova Southeastern University in 2002 with honors. Through her experience in the private and governmental sectors, she has also worked for law firms, corporations and for the Venezuelan Supreme Court of Justice.

FREDERICK VILLARI

Frederick Villari was born in Medfield, Massachusetts. He attended the University of Miami for his undergraduate degree in Business Law and History. He continued his education at Roger Williams University School of Law where he received his Juris Doctor. After passing the Florida Bar he embarked on his legal career to become an Assistant Attorney General for the Office of the Attorney General under Charlie Christ. Then he moved on in his legal career to the Miami-Dade County State Attorney's Office under Katherine Fernandez-Rundle and served as an Assistant State Attorney. He has finally found his home and family working for the Miami-Dade County Health Department Legal Office. He is currently licensed to practice law in Florida, New York and the District of Columbia. Moreover, Frederick is licensed in the Southern, Middle and Northern District of Florida Federal Bars. Frederick is happily married to Francesca and they have a two beautiful children, Erick and Alexa.

BEN ZIPKIN

Ben Zipken is a newly minted attorney in the state of Florida. He received a Bachelor of Science degree in Psychology from the University of Florida and a Juris Doctor from the University of Miami. Ben is working at the Department of Health on a fellowship grant and has thoroughly enjoyed his time with them.

Subscribe! Renew!
Give A Gift Of Health!

Give yourself or a friend or your favorite library, university or medical professional:

	Price	Quantity	Totals
Healthy Stories, Bonding Health with the Arts (2011)	$11.00	* _____	= $_____
Healthy Stories, America's Public Health Literary Journal (2010)	$11.00	* _____	= $_____
Healthy Stories, America's Award Winning Public Health Story Book (2009)	$11.00	* _____	= $_____
Healthy Stories, Sharing our Health Department Stories with the World (2008)	$11.00	* _____	= $_____
Healthy Stories, Did You Hear the Story about the Health Department That? (2007)	$11.00	* _____	= $_____

** Price includes shipping and handling.

TOTAL: = $_____

Send Healthy Stories to: Name:
Address:
City, State, Zip Code:

Send to:
Name:
Address:
City, State, Zip Code:

Send to:
Name:
Address:
City, State, Zip Code:

Please make checks payable to Miami-Dade County Health Department. Please send your order to:
Miami-Dade County Health Department
c/o Editor-in-Chief, Healthy Stories
8323 NW 12th Street, Suite 214
Miami, FL 33126

(786) 845-0300